The Body Alone

The Body Alone

A Lyrical Articulation of Chronic Pain

Nina Lohman

University of Iowa Press » Iowa City

University of Iowa Press, Iowa City 52242
Copyright © 2024 by Nina Lohman
uipress.uiowa.edu
Printed in the United States of America

Cover design by Kathleen Lynch
Text design and typesetting by Sara T. Sauers
Printed on acid-free paper

Library of Congress Cataloging-in-Publication Data
Names: Lohman, Nina, author.
Title: The Body Alone: A Lyrical Articulation of Chronic Pain /
Nina Lohman.
Description: Iowa City: University of Iowa Press, [2024]
Identifiers: LCCN 2023045667 (print) | LCCN 2023045668 (ebook) |
ISBN 9781609389499 (paperback) | ISBN 9781609389505 (ebook)
Subjects: LCSH: Chronic pain. | Chronic pain—Treatment.
Classification: LCC RB127.5.C48 L64 2024 (print) |
LCC RB127.5.C48 (ebook) | DDC 616/.0472—dc23/eng/20231222
LC record available at https://lccn.loc.gov/2023045667
LC ebook record available at https://lccn.loc.gov/2023045668

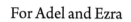

For Adel and Ezra

« *The body is not mute, but it is inarticulate.* »

—ARTHUR W. FRANK

<< >>

A NURSE IN GREEN SCRUBS ARRIVES AT MY BEDSIDE, his rubber-soled shoes squeaking against the linoleum floor. He holds out a pillow, instructing me to place it between my knees, *roll onto your side and pull your knees to your chest, yes, like that, now hold your shins.* Fluorescent light overhead mocks the faded plaster; even the facade of this place is sick. A patched wall as a premonition. *Hold that position— the doctor will be here soon.*

The man in the bed next to me does not speak. He wears a prison-issued orange jumpsuit. His wrists are handcuffed to the side rails of the bed and I hear the drag of metal on metal as he tries to move. Two police officers, motionless sentinels, stand quietly at his side. Their presence makes me nervous.

Paper pulled quickly from the back of a plastic container, the nauseating smell of latex, the snap of a glove as the doctor pulls it over his fingers, releasing it across his wrist. He is young. He is almost handsome. He is rushed. *Hold still,* he says, untying the drawstring on my paper gown. *You will feel the needle go into your spine. I need you to hold completely still.*

Why does no one paint this wall? Why are the lights so bright? What is the opposite of a talisman? *Tuck your chin.*

Lumbar Puncture Instructions for Beginners

Use the skin swabs and antiseptic solution to clean the skin in a circular fashion, starting at the L3–L4 interspace and moving outward to include at least one interspace above and one below. Just before applying the skin swabs, warn the patient that the solution is very cold; application of an unexpectedly cold solution can be unnerving for the patient.

He pushes the needle surely until it breaks the skin and enters the spinal canal, a casual move that rewrites history. In the shadow of my fetal pose the object he holds appears delicate, incapable of harm.

I should know better. Things are rarely as they seem.

As if to balance some requisite internal scale, I feel my limbs grow heavy as the needle draws fluid from the center of my spine. This compensated weight grounds my curved body to the bed, immobilizing my already compromised posture. He no longer instructs me to hold still, for I have become more statue than woman. What if our metaphors are all wrong and death is less like rising to the heavens and more like rooting to the core of the earth?

What matters is this: a needle rips a hole in my spine and I let it happen. As instructed, I hold my knees tight against my chest and tuck my chin, exposing the vulnerable curve of my back to a man whose name I don't even know.

This is the day pain becomes resident inside me. The moment when everything changes because it is when my body breaks clean in half, a rift that still echoes when I yell into it.

The problem with this story is that it has never been entirely clear where it might go.

This complicates the telling.

You see, it's not exactly linear. My story, like pain itself, swivels erratically—often without any warning at all. You'll need to pay close attention to keep up. It loops back right when you expect it to tumble forward. It pauses unpredictably then stays in the same place, stunted and sweaty, awkwardly, sometimes you won't believe how long it is possible for one thing to sit in the same place, but it does, stuck, oh my god we are still here, stuck, for far too long. I'll need you to be patient. The chronology of pain is circuitous.

In telling this story, there will be times when language collapses entirely into opaqueness. The tone will dislocate itself. Stay with me when this happens. *We tell ourselves stories in order to live.* Yes, this is true, but not all stories lend themselves to telling. Some actively resist our attempts at communication. And even when we do manage to coerce the words out of our mouths and into the world, or, in my case, onto the page, sometimes it takes more than one try to get the story right.

When it comes to stories, we like the ones where A leads to B and B leads to C. This arc is familiar, and familiarity inspires in us a sense of control. Remember this, you will want to return to it later: never underestimate the importance of control. Absent predictability, we crave assurance that stories, those alchemic tellings and retellings of our lives, will arrive at proper and resolute endings. Or, at the very least, that they will render crisp life lessons, knowledge that will properly equip us to better understand something new about ourselves and our place in this complicated world.

Otherwise, what's the point, right?

Because here's the thing: We desperately want it all to mean something, don't we? Of course we do. Without meaning, the brokenness of life is senseless and random. The unimaginable is coming for us and for those we hold most dear. So to protect ourselves and those we love, we isolate destruction, we do our best to wall off failure and pain so that we can imbue it with meaning. We summon a reason for its arrival, a purpose for its stay; we observe a course it must take. When we supply meaning, we lessen the fixed sting of pain. We steel ourselves against the brokenness of our bodies and the world we inhabit. We secure necessary space between our most vulnerable selves and life's undeniable shortcomings. That's why, when we can scaffold meaning onto a broken situation, we discover a peculiar sense of agency over chaos. We tell ourselves stories not only to live but because stories give meaning to our pain and that pain means something can be endured.

So how do you tell a story where A does not lead to B because instead A leads to mint tea then to fireflies above a lake then eventually A finds its way to C and don't worry B does arrive but not until the very end? Forget telling. I want to know: How do you live a life that riddles this way? How do you extract meaning from a story that refuses to hold still?

I crave a clean origin. One I can point my finger at and say with conviction, *right here—this is the starting point.* But it just so happens that this is not a reality from which I get to choose. I wasn't given control over this part of the story. That's okay. We'll make do. In place of certainty, I claim this as the beginning: I woke on a cold January morning with an ache like a bruise spreading across the left side of my head.

On the day the pain began, I thought little of its intrusion in my life. I attributed it to overexertion, to hours spent slumped in poor posture reading and writing my way through graduate school. I had just completed an arduous class cycle and figured this pain, this headache, was my body's way of coming down off the high stress load I had been carrying. I was probably getting sick. Maybe I had the flu.

Headaches were unusual for me. They weren't my body's typical response to overstimulation and when they did arrive, they were never cause for alarm. They were minor upsets solved by a couple over-the-counter pills and extra water. Rest.

I did little but lie on the couch, waiting for the pain to subside on its own. I watched bad daytime TV, my body curled under a down blanket on the too-small vintage leather couch in the basement. I slept then woke, I may have even taken a few ibuprofens, but the pain refused to budge. Instead, it grew worse as the day progressed. When the sun eventually dipped behind the rugged mountain peak, fear spread like a hot, alarming pulse beating just below the surface of my skin. I was unnervingly alert, begging my body to proffer clues as to what was wrong and how I could possibly fix it. Was I having a stroke? What does dying feel like? Does it feel like being absorbed by your own body? I sat still, accounting for each breath, insecure yet somehow cognizant that each passing moment was ferrying me away from that elusive physical sensation so often defined only by its absence: normal.

This was no ordinary headache. This was a call demanding a response.

We threaded our arms through winter coats, stuffed our feet into snow boots—not bothering with the laces—and drove to the closest emergency room. I sat rigid in a plastic chair, cold air whipping into the waiting room each time the double glass doors retracted, announcing the arrival of newcomers. Once admitted, my legs shook with an adrenaline-fueled tremor I could not control as the triage nurse, a woman with thin wrists and long, strong fingers, took my temperature, my blood pressure, my pulse. She asked my age and wondered if I smoked and did anyone in my family have a history of stroke?

27. No. Yes.

I should tell you now, this is a story that doesn't end well.

Or maybe it's better to say that this is a story that doesn't end how you think it will end.

Or maybe I should just tell it to you exactly like it is: this is a story that doesn't end.

Tuck your chin.

A needle rips a hole in my spine, forcing cerebrospinal fluid to drip into a narrow plastic vial. *It's not cloudy—that's a good sign.* Necessary nothingness mined from the core of my being. *Not bloody, either.* A plexus of cells hatched in the deep ventricles of my brain scrutinized by a third-shift ER doctor. *Almost done here.*

A band of orderlies appear at the bedside of the man in the orange jumpsuit. With the wordless, practiced ease of professionals, they release the foot brakes holding the bed in place. Their feet shuffle, someone sighs loudly, the bed creaks as it is pushed into the narrow hallway. Because I am curled toward the wall and away from the center of the room, I only hear the movement behind my back. At the door, I watch as the orderly, the nurse, then the man in the bed exit the room.

For the briefest of moments, the man in the orange jumpsuit and I share a common vulnerability: our compromised mobility forces us to rely on the knowledge, compassion, and skill of other people. I am at the same time relieved and ashamed of my relief as his bed is wheeled away. I had been afraid that the man would, for some reason, spontaneously react, causing an altercation in the already cramped room. I had convinced myself that should this happen, in the swell of commotion, the Almost Handsome Physician would be bumped and the needle in my spine would twist and puncture and paralyze.

The police officers are the last to leave the room as though indicating the end of a parade. Or a funeral.

It's difficult to understand the pain of other people.

Especially when not everyone's voice is heard.

I doubt his story ends well either.

These are the words: patients are advised to remain horizontal for a minimum of three hours post-procedure for the punctured dura mater surrounding the spinal cord to begin the process of healing. Most of the time, a blood clot will form, thereby stopping the cerebrospinal fluid leak and reestablishing proper equilibrium.

This is the experience: the consequence of insufficient cerebral pressure is the rearrangement of prescribed gravity inside your body. What was once grounded is now unsinkable. Pull and push and settle refuse the curvature of uneven mass. You hear sounds that exist solely inside the echo of your frame. The bed where you rest is your event horizon, beyond which there is no escape.

Doctors call this a spinal headache. Such a tidy term for tumult.

Night becomes morning as we are led to a windowless room to wait for the lab results. The pain that sent me to the hospital—a singular headache from an unknown source, what felt like a bruise spreading across the left side of my head—is now compounded by a headache from the lumbar puncture. This newest headache feels like the downbeat of a heavy pulse, like soreness flexing its muscles, like a depressurizing of my spine. I never knew it was possible to have more than one type of headache at the same time.

I went to the hospital assuming the doctors would eliminate the pain. I believed the hierarchy of medicine would justify itself and I would be rid of my affliction. I assumed that when the double glass doors retracted and I walked into the emergency room on that January night, the doctors I met would swiftly cipher the pain from my body.

I am embarrassed by the privilege and naivety this thought pattern reveals. That I lacked the capacity to entertain an alternative proves how deeply engrained this thinking, this worldview, at the time, was.

What happened that night in the emergency room was this: I was treated with respect, care, dignity, and swiftness by health care professionals.

What happened that night in the emergency room was also this: no one knew what to do with me.

Instead of eliminating the pain, that night it was made worse. What began as a single, though spreading, deep, dull ache gnarled itself into a tender knot of wounds. I went to the hospital expecting a diagnosis followed by a treatment plan. I wanted relief. I wanted to be transformed into a readable document, a line of numbers and letters that could be easily defined. I sought assurance from someone whose job it is to know how bodies work to tell me that my body would be just fine. *Here*, I thought they might say, *don't be afraid. Take this. You'll be better by morning.*

I should have known better.

Things are rarely as they seem.

From the bowels of the hospital, the radiologist evaluates the CT scans, confirming a healthy, functioning brain with no bleeds or masses. A lab technician draws results from the lumbar puncture to conclusively eliminate meningitis. The blood panel suggests no elevated levels of concern. I have no injury, illness, or infection. What I have, they tell me, is a symptom. What I have is pain without source or end.

The Almost Handsome Physician tells me his shift has ended. He prints a pamphlet on cluster headaches, scribbles a prescription for Valium, and tells me to follow up with my primary care physician in a week. He clicks the end of his pen, the tip retracting quickly into the barrel. *Rest and be sure to drink lots of fluids,* he says before walking out the door.

There are things you should know.

You see, I was healthy until, quite suddenly, one day I was not. Susan Sontag describes it like this: *Everyone who is born holds dual citizenship, in the kingdom of the well and in the kingdom of the sick. Although we all prefer to use only the good passport, sooner or later each of us is obliged, at least for a spell, to identify ourselves as citizens of that other place.*

Citizenship. The kingdom of the well and the kingdom of the sick. Passports. Place. Obligation and identification. These familiar words are signposts designed to help us find the ground beneath our feet. It's no wonder that illness narratives, the stories people tell about their encounters with sickness, return again and again to Sontag's metaphor. In illness, we leave behind one land to become citizens of another. It's remarkable how easy it is to slip into metaphors when trying to explain the unknown. It's tempting to stop right there.

But Sontag continues and so must we.

My point is that illness is not *a metaphor, and that the most truthful way of regarding illness—and the healthiest way of being ill—is one most purified of, most resistant to, metaphoric thinking.*

I am interested in knowing *the healthiest way of being ill.*

I am interested in using metaphor, in using language, not to replace knowledge but to fill in its gaps.

Before the rift split me open, before the needle slid into my spine, even before the ache like a bruise that sent me to the hospital in the first place, I lived comfortably in the kingdom of the well. My body responded to commands. It recovered. It generated. It welcomed. My bones maintained the precise, smooth architecture of their original creation. I slept.

I experienced pain like most people do—in fleeting moments anchored to a direct cause. Pain was circumstantial. It was acute. When it arrived, it did so as one piece of a much larger picture. I could draw a line between action and consequence: a fall resulted in a scabbed knee, extra laps in the pool constricted the muscles in my shoulders. These actions produced knowable pains in my body. I never had to search for their meaning. Also—and this is a distinction that matters—at some point the pain would end. My body would right itself once again and stasis would be restored, ordinary function would resume.

I grew up strong and athletic. I was a swimmer with toned shoulders and a powerful kick. I logged hours, years, in the community swimming pool pulling my body back and forth across the lanes while coaches paced across the slippery deck, chlorine and salt layered constantly on my skin, my hair brittle, shiny, perpetually damaged. As an athlete, I was familiar with the practice of pushing through pain to achieve goals. Pain was proof: proof of discipline, proof I was getting better, closer, stronger. Pain was an obstacle I worked to overcome. It was a force I aimed to dominate through sheer strength and stubborn will. This version of pain is culturally acceptable and encouraged. Like the varsity stripes on my letterman jacket, I wore it proudly as a badge.

But then, without warning or cause, in my mid-twenties and otherwise healthy, I woke in the kingdom of the sick with an ache like a bruise spreading across the left side of my head. In both location and intensity, the pain was unfamiliar. It identified equally as sharp and dull, as intimate and other. It spoke in a language I could not understand.

No. That's not how it happened.

Illness is not a metaphor.

There was no language and it was not speaking and I understood how it all might end. What happened was this: there was a physical response (pain) to a stimulus (unknown) that produced within my body an emotional reaction (fear).

I don't think I'm writing all this merely to discover *the healthiest way of being ill*. I think there's a much larger truth I'm trying to uncover.

When the pain began, I was a second-year graduate student studying stories. Theology, specifically. Because *we tell ourselves stories in order to live*, remember? Because we desperately want it all to mean something, don't we? The sweeping narrative of theology, its language in particular, captivated me.

I didn't grow up in a church. I arrived at theology through my own choosing in my late teens, free from familial and institutional indoctrination. Where other children were taught the miracle of Jesus feeding crowds with a few loaves of bread and some small fish, I was read bedtime stories about Athena springing forth from Zeus's head. I was a quiet, strange child who was often lost in the stories that unfolded inside my mind. I struggled in school, especially, ironically, with reading and writing, but I readily and often fabricated imaginary worlds and scenarios within my head. I dreamt vivid dreams, the texture and details of which I can to this day still recall. There was nothing I loved more than creating entire worlds inside of dollhouses, tree houses, piles of snow, closets, LEGO creations, and forts.

When I was young, my family had this big yellow book of Greek myths. I would spend hours staring at the graphics, often violent drawings of gods exacting revenge on mortals, of rowdy centaurs and crafty harp-strumming muses. The stories themselves were explicit, at times difficult to follow, equal parts frightening and intriguing. The myths taught me to trace the origins of everyday mysteries back to ancient texts. Each story contained a complete explanation for an absurd situation—a reason, however bizarre, that explained the outcome. *Nothing was left of Echo but her voice, which to this day can be heard senselessly repeating the words of others.* Through these stories, I learned that actions beget consequences. *The moment she opened the lid, out swarmed a horde of miseries: Greed, Vanity, Slander, Envy, and all the evils that until then had been unknown to mankind.* I learned punishment. *At night his immortal liver grew anew, but every day the eagle returned and he had to suffer again.*

I learned words that stretched simple emotions sideways—words like gloom and vulgar, scorn and gaiety.

Though I was young, I understood myths were stories, not truths, and yet something about them made sense to me. I was the kind of kid who gravitated toward stories that promised morals and clean takeaways. What I appreciated about them was how they collapsed enormity into the obvious. They made the unknowable tangible.

It's no wonder I eventually found my way to theology. Like the myths of my childhood, theology told stories through images of light and dark, joy and love and anger. Like myths, these stories were centered on generations of families wherein the act of storytelling was an important feature of the story itself. I understood how the discipline tried to provide, both historically but also to the contemporary reader, context for the chaotic, hurtful world.

Because I was raised on Zeus, not Jesus, when I began to study theology, the text was fresh and had something to teach. I was able to dwell inside the seemingly endless debates of origin, meaning, and application without having to undo denominational doctrines rooted in my childhood. Though I lacked the absolute faith of my ordination-bound classmates, I possessed the raw curiosity of an outsider. I didn't mind this distinction; I could hold my own, a skill that proved useful when situations grew tense in class debates. I was able to keep my calm because I never felt like the core of my existence was threatened when I was pressed by conservative professors and even more conservative classmates.

Theology is not the same as religion, nor is it synonymous with Christianity, though the study historically has leaned heavily on the tradition of many noted Christian thinkers. Theology is an academic study concerned with the nature of the divine and the practice of religious beliefs. Though there are theologians who are Christians, there are also those who are not. Religious observation is no more a requisite for theology than a lab coat is required for science. It may help you to look the part, it may offer protection, but it's certainly not the garment that qualifies the laborer for the work.

I will admit that while I was drawn to theology in large part because of the text itself, there were pieces of my own belief system and worldview with which I felt compelled to reckon. As a young adult, I had crafted within myself something that looked like belief, or at least I hoped very much for it to assume the shape of belief. I wanted to believe in God. I did. Sincerely. I had this notion that everything would be easier if I believed because faith would provide both a community and a rubric for navigating life, two qualities that as a secular loner of sorts, I craved. I wanted to claim as true the stories I heard about struggle and provision. I wanted the grace and stability that I saw in those around me whose commitments oriented around their beliefs. I wanted my life, my struggles, to mean something. There was a longing in me eager to believe there was more to life than what I could see.

As a teenager, I began to attend youth groups where I was taught to pray. I followed suit, all the while desperately trying to configure what was inside of me into a belief in the divine. But the truth is that I was more taken by social acceptance than I was by the message of Christianity. It's possible that this is where I first learned to disassociate my internal experience from my external one, which is another way of saying that I've never been very good at aligning the person I am on the inside with the person I am on the outside. Articulating truth is a vulnerable exercise for anyone, but especially so for an awkward teenage girl. Still, for several years as a late teen, I tried to believe in God, but there was always a deep and unrelenting snag, in me or in the fundamental construct of faith, I could never entirely tell which, that kept me at a distance and rendered full immersion impossible.

As quickly as it formed, my budding faith dissolved. Yet, oddly, my theological curiosity remained. In college, I studied English and geography because I was interested in how place shaped people and the stories they told. The intersection of geography, story, and religion felt like fertile academic ground to pursue.

I enrolled in graduate school to study theology, wherein I learned its place in history, its authorship and audience. I traced its meandering stories from beginning to end. I studied Greek so that I could read the original text. I came to know what was omitted, what was argued out, what was questionable, what was nuanced, what was gendered, what was contextual. I allowed myself to get lost in its poetic beauty. I cried at the raw heartbreak of the laments.

I was an inquisitive student. I was happy. I was married. At the time, he and I lived in Colorado. We bought our first house, a tiny pale stucco that sat on the corner lot of a double-wide street, and assigned a place to each item we owned. I liked it best when the windows were open, the sheer curtains billowing like sails. I created an office of heavy textbooks, a cumbersome desktop computer, pictures of loves far away. He would bring me mugs of steaming coffee while I worked. In the backyard, branches of a mature crab apple dangled like fringe. We had no pets or children. That first Colorado spring, we planted a vegetable garden in the empty lot behind the garage. I would often break from studying to walk the narrow rows, the idle task of pulling weeds a welcome reprieve. We walked the neighborhood, always talking, hand in hand. We listened to the radio as we made dinner. We drove to see family in Iowa for Christmas.

Upon purchase, the realtor called ours a *first and last neighborhood*, a somber but accurate epitaph. Our neighbors were Howard and Corrine, Barbara and Herald. We sat cordially in their overly warm living rooms on dated but pristine furniture drinking weak coffee. We would check in when the weather was inclement. Herald and Barbara drove their motor home to Arizona for the winter. Howard and Corrine walked the same routes at the same times every day. Once we helped decorate a Christmas tree. To the west, mountains, almost always a trace of snow on the peak.

Ask yourself this question: How much pain can you handle?

He clicks the end of his pen, the tip retracting quickly into the barrel. *Rest and be sure to drink lots of fluids*, he says before walking out the door.

I don't remember leaving the hospital. I don't remember if I sat in the front of the car or if I laid across the back seat. I don't remember walking through the snow and into the pale-yellow house. I don't remember kicking off my boots. I don't remember sleeping. I don't remember that night. Or the morning that followed.

When I wake, I hear movement in the kitchen. That means I slept. That means the Valium worked. Those who say they want to lie in bed all day are those who have never been forced to lie in bed all day. Flat on my back, staring at the ceiling, I can distinguish between the parts of my head that ache like a bruise—the original pain—and the parts that reverberate like a hollow drum—the consequence of the lumbar puncture that has yet to heal. There are layers to this headache. Valium, the first lick of opioid in my system, helps me sleep but does nothing to quell the pain.

He is cooking dinner in the kitchen, but eating requires the unthinkable task of raising my head above the horizontal plane of the bed. To assuage boredom while fending off hunger, I try moving without actually moving. I extend my left arm to the bedside table feeling for the radio. As though reading braille, my fingers recognize the raised indentation of the power button. To turn it on I will need to rotate my shoulder.

Pause.

I should know better. Even children know better.

Remember when we were little? How we would dance and sing the song about the skeleton? *The hip bone's connected to the backbone. The backbone's connected to the neck bone.*

My backbone is, currently, leaking.

I lie motionless but for the colossal effort of staying alive. Pipes bring water to the kitchen sink. To turn the radio on I will have to move by actually moving. This requires shifting onto my left side and reaching my right arm across my body. I hold my breath, moving in centimeters, not inches. Still, I feel the gravel below the boulder begin to slip.

No. That's not how it happened.

What I am actually feeling, the sensation responsible for the pain that feels like a hollow drum, is my brain pressing against the nerves on the edge of my skull.

Pause again.

Hold this position. Wait. Now, once more: move. My finger finds the switch. *Our show today in three acts. Act One, It's Not a Crack House, It's a Crack Home, in which we see what happens when bad houses happen to good people.*

Vocabulary Lessons

Paradox:

(noun) A statement or tenet contrary to received opinion or belief, especially one that is difficult to believe. Of multiple origins. Partly a borrowing from French. Partly a borrowing from Latin and Greek, παρα- ("para-") + δόξα ("opinion").

Used in a sentence:

I am entirely healthy, I am entirely in pain; an incessant contradiction, I am nothing if not a paradox.

The first winter of pain becomes the first spring of pain. Already it's been four months since the headache began. No one—not the doctors, not the shaman in the mountains, not the chiropractor, not even my own mother—knows what to do.

The dura surrounding the leaking hole in my spine eventually closes, weeks and weeks after they said it would, reestablishing a necessary wall between the liquid designed to cushion my brain and everything else that exists under the sun. With this barrier of membrane comes slight relief. Now I have only one version of pain—the original one—to deal with. Sitting becomes standing becomes walking. Next the laundry then a movie until finally I am strong enough to resume my studies. But health is more of a charade than an identity. A functioning body ought not to be confused with wellness.

Things are rarely as they seem.

Little pinch.

The vein bulges blue below the rubber tourniquet as the medical assistant, a woman with a gentle smile, slips the needle into my antecubital fossa, injecting lustrous purple-black liquid metal under my skin. *Try not to move.* The magnetic pull of teslas. The alignment of molecules in a private field inside this body but beyond my view.

The iodine contrasts a functioning system without visible impairment. Only when seeking an elusive diagnosis is health the wrong answer.

Try not to move. I walk the aisles of the grocery store, pain boring into the sides of my head. Try not to move. I sink into the tub, the water hot, my skin instantly red, pain boring into the sides of my head. Try not to move. I sweep the kitchen floor, pain boring into the sides of my head. Try not to move. He kisses the back of my neck. Try not to move. I can't sleep. Try not to move.

Needles push drugs in. Needles pull blood out. I swallow pills in the morning, pills with lunch, pills in the evening before I toss and turn all night in bed. I pay for chiropractic adjustments to my spine. I lie naked, covered only by a thin sheet, waiting for a massage. I lie naked, covered only by a thin sheet, waiting for acupuncture. I hold still, trying not to breathe as the MRI machine clanks and bangs inches above my head. I drive through the mountains to the neighboring town to visit a healer who tells me to throw out any food in my refrigerator that is more than three days old.

Nothing I do or ingest or release eases the pain.

I understand that illness is not a metaphor, but what other tools do I have to communicate? This experience is like throwing pebbles at a massive wall hoping it will crack. I long to create a fissure large enough to crawl through so I can rejoin the land of the well, the land I recognize as home. The ground at my feet is littered with my feeble attempts. But the wall doesn't budge. Of course it doesn't. My efforts do little more than expose my desperation.

This experience has launched me into a new space. What Sontag neglected to mention is that between the kingdom of the well and the kingdom of the sick there exists a no-woman's-land. It's a distinct territory, a dusty blot on the map, a place defined by its borders.

I live here now. I am a citizen of in-between.

I can function, mostly. I am normal, mostly. I'm just in near-constant pain. Waiting rooms are full of women like me, fellow citizens of the land of in-between. We are not exactly sick, but we certainly are not healthy, either. You might recognize us by the shadow in the back of our eyes. We look as tired as we feel. Would you mind turning down the music just a bit? Yes, the lights, too. You've seen us, haven't you? We are your sister. Your neighbor. The woman in the office next door. We are your mother. We are your wife. Your daughter. The meaninglessness of our pain confounds the disorder we constantly endure.

We, the women of in-between, are expert travelers. Sometimes we exist in the kingdom of the well and those are wonderful days. On these days we make plans and we initiate outings. Our convictions align with our efforts. We are productive. We think *maybe*. We buy plants for the garden; we fully intend to dig into the waiting earth. Other times we exist in the kingdom of the sick. On those days, we conserve our energy because we need it to survive. We nestle into the corner of the couch. We send texts that begin with, *I'm sorry, but* . . . We watch the dishes pile haphazardly in the sink. We press our fingertips against our tender spots. But sometimes, perhaps even most of the time, we have the opportunity to stand with one foot firmly in each kingdom. In these moments, we are alchemists harnessing the power of our otherness to transform this tangled, unchosen existence.

We are in-between. Neither sick nor healthy. Both sick and healthy.

We are undiagnosed. We are underdiagnosed. We are wrongly diagnosed. Our bodies resist the known categories of disease. Our pain is unstoppable. We are mysteries. We are unbelievable.

Because that's what we are told by every physician, every clinician, every well-intentioned passerby and friend of a friend: the pain in our bodies, the untraceable, incurable, cyclical, unknowable—*Is it even real? She sure doesn't act like she's in pain. Are you sure you aren't just depressed? My aunt had something like that but after menopause it all went away. There's always something wrong with her, isn't there? If I hurt as much as she says she does, then I wouldn't be here tonight.*—it doesn't mean anything. It just is and no one seems to know why. If we can't see it or trace it or measure it, if we can't cure it, if it isn't actually killing you, then we are sorry, but we don't know what to do with you.

Take it easy.

It's probably just stress.

In a way this new territory where I find myself, the land of in-between, makes perfect sense. I have never been one to fit in. I am an almost-but-not-quite in nearly every category. A margin dweller. A Tuesday girl in a Friday world. These days, I look healthy and by most accounts I am healthy. I no longer carry the hollow pain from the botched spinal tap and yet there remains in every moment of every day an inflexible pain in my body—headache, yes, but it is more broad and deep than an ache.

Ache. What a careless word for a sensation with the power to dismantle a life.

Clinical Documentation

The patient has already been to a chiropractor and acupuncturist with no results. She used to run but has not been running because she is afraid of the headaches. I encouraged her to resume her running program slowly, that she obtain massage therapy for fifteen minutes three to four times a week, and that she do yoga and progressive relaxation techniques. I reassured her that at this point she has had so much evaluation that I doubt that there is anything seriously wrong, and that she may have started with a musculoskeletal pain that seems to have just increased and not gone away for several months.

I break from studying where I am immersed in systematic theology, which, as the name suggests, is an ordered approach to the biblical narrative. I enjoy this categorization of doctrine. (Margin dweller.) As I read, I underline the words of the German theologian Paul Tillich. *It is impossible to speak of being without also speaking of becoming. What does experience by participation reveal? For that which concerns us ultimately must belong to reality as a whole.*

I rise from my chair, lace my fingers together above my head, stretching tall. My arms arc wide as I lower them to my sides, stacking my hands on my hips, extending my neck left then right. I exhale. Idly, my right hand slides under my shirt to the small of my back where fibrous scar tissue lines my spine like graffiti. This invisible tag irritates me. Minor degrees of variance, like when I lean against the rim of the sink to wash my hands, make it feel as though unyielding tectonic plates are compressing my spine.

Our ultimate concern is that which determines our being or non-being.

Something is amiss inside my body and I need to know why. There is a blue ache that for months has lodged itself in my body. It is resident, untouched by effort or will. But why? Where did it come from and what will make it go away? What does this kind of pain mean? The doctors I have seen assure me that the presenting symptom—the pain in my head—is indicative of a greater problem; it is not in and of itself the problem. Symptoms, such as headaches and pain, are clues to follow. They are road maps that will guide us to the real issue; they are not themselves the destination.

I settle back into my desk chair, exhale once more, opening the book to the earmarked page.

A clue. A road map. A fibrous scar.

Every part is dependent on every other part.

Paul Tillich was removed from his professorship at the University of Frankfurt by Adolf Hitler in 1933. He is known for a method of correlation that aligns insights from Christian revelation with issues raised by existential, psychological, and philosophical analysis. In other words, he believed, more or less, in a Möbius strip of questions and answers.

Nothing can be of ultimate concern for us which does not have the power of threatening and saving our being.

Tillich's approach—systematic theology as a whole—makes sense to me. I can see the benefit of cataloging life this way. I can see how placing these insights side by side can offer cohesion to what otherwise seems chaotic. I understand the urge to find the role of the individual housed inside the experience of the corporate. I am curious as to how the privateness of pain parallels the privateness of belief.

An invisible tag. A call demanding a response. A rift that still echoes.

Providence is a paradoxical concept.

Vocabulary Lessons

Providence:

(noun) Foresight; anticipation of and preparation for the future; prudent management, government, or guidance. Of multiple origins. Partly a borrowing from French. Partly a borrowing from the Latin *provident*, which is the present participle of *prōvidēre*, meaning "provide" + *-ia*.

Used in a sentence:

I see no providence here.

Consistency: An Inventory

Each new day is the same as the one before.

Prometheus's liver regenerated nightly.

Pain settles above my ears, bilaterally, reaching forward to my temples, pulling the muscles behind my eyes, spreading like eager rivulets across my forehead, reaching down to the base of my skull, pooling in the suboccipital triangle, draining down my neck, settling in my shoulders. When I wake in the morning, I wake in pain. When I sit at my desk, when I drink red wine, when I laugh, when he lifts my shirt over my head and pulls me to bed, all of it filters through pain.

He

He tells me he doesn't mind sitting in the waiting rooms. He'll bring a book or read a magazine. He holds my hand as we walk in the crisp mountain air, slowly, silently, around the block. He says it doesn't make sense to him, either. He says it's okay that I can't do as much as I used to be able to do. He says it won't always be this way.

Vocabulary Lessons

_____:

(adjective) I want a word for the melodic sequence of cracks and pops that emit from the bones in my hand, my wrist, my shoulder as I reach back to knead the taut muscle at the base of my neck.

The word is orange. It would be plastic. There's a satisfaction to saying the word correctly but please note you can only say it while exhaling, not inhaling. It will make you think of marbles and tails. Apple blossoms. The word ends as quickly as it begins; it may feel a bit like wicker.

Used in a sentence:
Darling, come closer to me, I know you are hurting, I just heard _____ from across the room.

Prescription

The pharmacist has stapled the directions to the outside of the paper bag. I pull the staple loose, shaking the plastic bottle into my hand, then twist off the lid to reveal a heap of small round tablets. They are yellow but the hue of the bottle causes them to appear green. I replace the lid, twisting right until it clicks back into place, then set the bottle on the counter.

As I pull the pamphlet free from the bag, my finger catches the edge of the twisted staple. Reflexively, I put the tip of my finger in my mouth, sucking away the blood that rises to the surface. I recently started seeing a new general practitioner at the family medicine clinic not far from my home. She is a slip of a woman with a New York accent. I like her; therefore, I readily try the medications she prescribes.

Pamphlet in hand, I scan the list of possible side effects: *dizziness, drowsiness, anxiety, insomnia, strange dreams, dry mouth, stuffy nose, blurred vision, constipation, breast swelling, missed menstrual periods, weight gain, swelling in hands or feet, impotence, trouble having an orgasm, mild itching, skin rash, headache, low blood pressure.*

Acne medication when I was a teenager and birth control have, until now, been the only medications I have taken with regularity. I feel my pulse quicken as I read the prescribed uses: *antipsychotic and antiemetic. Can treat nausea and vomiting. It can also treat anxiety and schizophrenia.*

How did this happen? How did I get to a place where I am being prescribed antipsychotics? I have headaches. There is a pain in my head but the pain is not *in* my head. I am not psychotic.

Am I?

Prescription

Dutifully, as instructed by both pharmacist and physician, each morning I swallow a yellow pill alongside my breakfast. Once it enters my bloodstream, the medicine makes my brain feel fuzzy, as though a scrim has been erected between my thoughts and my words. I can almost feel it as it descends like the curtain on a stage. It drops right down the middle of my brain, a gauzy veil that hinders my attempt to retrieve words. It's fitting, yes? I am a woman divided. The pain, resident on both sides of the scrim, resilient as ever, untouched.

It's Not: An Inventory

It's not in my hair or my nose or my elbow, forearm, or wrist.
My fingernails are fine. I can still crack my knuckles like a bored
schoolgirl waiting for the bell. It's not in my breasts, it does not
pull at my sternum; generally my abdomen and belly button are
just fine. My ribs hold ground without protest. The small of my
back curves appropriately, you will not find it hiding there, but
please let your hand linger in that space, I like how it makes me
feel. My hip bones, sit bones, femurs do not hurt; nor do my knees,
my shins, my ankles, my heels, my toes.

Providence is a paradoxical concept.

Clinical Documentation

Ms. Lohman is a right-handed woman who was evaluated today for headaches that began to occur in January of 2007. In describing the headaches, Ms. Lohman says they are bilateral and are felt strongest on the left side. The quality of the head pain is constant and pressure-like. Ms. Lohman estimates the maximal intensity of her headache to be 7 out of 10.

There is no intracranial hemorrhage, shift of the midline structures, mass or mass effect. No extra-axial fluid or hemorrhage identified. The skull and skull base appear intact. The visualized paranasal sinuses and mastoid air cells appear well aerated bilaterally.

At all cervical levels, the discs are normal in height without evidence of desiccation, bulge, or herniation. The neural foramina are patent and exiting nerve roots are intact. There is no evidence of spinal canal stenosis or narrowing. The posterior elements are intact. There is no evidence of mass.

On exam, she was in no acute distress. Pulse was 82 and blood pressure 121/73. Heart was at regular rhythm and rate.

Pain forces change.

The first spring of pain becomes the first summer of pain. I write my final paper, completing my graduate work in theology. Life in the mountains, once emblematic of independence and ripe with the promise of adventure, now feels isolating. Distant. It is a place imprinted with a time stamp marking the point where everything shifted. Graduate school was supposed to launch me into a career; a life of books and papers, of steady inquiry and rousing theological debate, or at the very least, people and conversation. But I don't launch. Instead, I lose. I lose any forward momentum I had generated. I lose contact with professors and peers. I lose the life that would have allowed me to study the intersection of literature and place and theology.

Instead of expanding outward, my life contracts. In many ways, this is an appropriate response to upheaval: smaller lives, by design, ought to be easier to protect, to predict. A smaller life should mean less stress, less uncertainty, less pain. I figure that if I can slow the activity, then there will be a chance I can identify the source of the pain. My focus is sharp—fix the problem, stop the pain; the rest of life will sort itself out in due time. I believe I will get better. I genuinely believe the pain both can and will end.

If there is a reason or an explanation for all of this, then I will find it. So I begin.

I eliminate all potential sources of pain. I quit my job. I pull back from volunteer commitments. I say no more than I say yes: to friends, to travel, to any activity that might possibly conflate the pain. Could it be environmental? Or allergens? I say yes to more appointments, to more doctors, clinics, to coffee with anyone with an idea of what might be wrong. Could it be my mattress? What about my glasses? Is the prescription correct? I should make an appointment with my optometrist to check.

Back in Iowa, where our families live, there is a pain clinic at a large, well-known hospital. There is a headache clinic. There is a neurology department where I can get outpatient treatment on a daily basis. This potential solution paired with the support from our families is enough to draw us out of the mountains and back to the Midwest.

It's an easy decision to make. For both of us. I want to do anything that I can to stop the pain and because he loves me, this is his wish as well. We sell the pale-yellow house, pack our belongings into the yawning cavern of a rented truck, and drive east to Iowa. I wasn't born in Iowa City, but it's where I was raised. It is where my parents, my sisters and their husbands, and my nieces and nephews all live. Now home, we sit around the table for Sunday dinners. We cheer from the sidelines at soccer games. Returning is both homecoming and failure—returning to Iowa this soon was never the plan.

We buy a modest redbrick home on a quiet street that was once the back curve of the county racetrack. The day we take possession of the home we sit on the floor of the porch, our backs resting against the wall, and open a bottle of champagne. We sip while wondering which spot in the backyard is best for the garden. I slip the cork into my pocket, wanting to remember the hope of the moment. We peel faded wallpaper from the bathroom, from the entryway, the living room. We paint the walls light French gray, the trim a crisp white. We pull back the carpet to discover pine hardwood floors in surprisingly good condition. In the backyard near the teetering fence the heavy blooms of white peonies bend recklessly at the neck.

If I can find the right combination of medicines, if we can narrow in on a diagnosis, if and when the pain begins to subside, it will be possible to create a pleasing life inside these new boundaries. I never assumed I would be anything but healthy in my life. How strange it is to define your identity by what you lack.

I will pivot.

I will see what else can give meaning to life.

If not school, if not a career, then maybe a family is possible.

Treatment Records: Two Years In

MEDICATIONS

Valium. Imitrex. Compazine. Dihydroergotamine (IV). Depacon
(IV). Reglan (IV). Prednisone. Zomig. Alprazolam. Topamax.
Duloxetine. Gabapentin. Cymbalta. Baclofen. Ibuprofen.

TESTS

Lumbar Puncture. CT Scan of Brain with Contrast. CT Scan of
Brain without Contrast. MRI Brain Scan. MRA Cerebral Scan.
CBC Blood Panel. Diabetes. Kidney. Liver. Thyroid Scan.
Heavy-Metal Screening. Celiac. Pregnancy. Urine.

SUPPLEMENTS

Vitamins D. Vitamin B_2. Vitamin B_{12}.

ALTERNATIVE TREATMENTS

Chiropractic Adjustments. Acupuncture. Reiki. Massage.
Therapy. Naturopathic Healing.

Lacking a diagnosis, all is suspect. Unknowing is an exhausting posture to maintain. *If you wish to make an apple pie from scratch, you must first invent the universe.* If you wish to eradicate the pain, you must first identify its source.

But how do you eradicate what remains invisible?

Begin with what it is you do know.

A few possibilities have been eliminated along the way. We know the source is not a tumor trapped in a recessed crease of my brain. I am not pregnant nor is it cancer or celiac. It doesn't present as migraine, either. Migraines are a different beast, one I'm grateful not to know. Though sudden, its arrival, I am told by every physician I meet, was not spontaneous. Pain doesn't just appear unbidden; it unfurls from a particular source.

Clinical Documentation

HISTORY OF PRESENT ILLNESS

Onset: Daily HA since 2007.

Location: Worse behind right eye o/w diffuse.

Severity: 9/10

Quality: Reports tingling sensation inside head. Pressure-like pain in occiput when lays down.

Timing: No trauma.

Context: Female with h/o daily headaches of unknown etiology started experiencing worsening headaches. Gradual increasing of tingling pain. She has been increasing her Neurontin dose for pain control. Has an appointment with PCP tomorrow.

Modifying factors: Neurontin does not improve pain.

Associated signs and symptoms: Lightheadedness and dizziness + ringing in ears + no vomiting. No recent illness or sick contacts + minimal neck stiffness but different from prior neck pain. No photophobia or phonophobia.

BP: 124/64

Pulse: 96

Resp: 18

Temperature: 35.5°C

Pain as a Vital Sign: A Primer

Medically speaking, pain is a response. It's what happens when stimulated nerves send a rush of messages designed to alert the brain of problems in the body. Think of it like a doorbell alerting you to the fact that someone is standing at your front door. The toll of the bell isn't the message; it's what alerts you to the fact that there is a message. In a similar way, pain is a signal (a doorbell), not a source (the person waiting at your front door).

For a while, pain, much like blood pressure and pulse, was considered a vital sign, a means of detection, a reflection of the body's essential function. Though pain is necessary in its own right—it's a sorry soul who is forced to live her short life absent this valuable warning system—the designation of pain as a vital sign was well intentioned but ultimately misguided.

The problem with classifying pain as a vital sign has less to do with function and more to do with measurement. While the intensity of pain can be measured externally through sliding scales and reported accounts of perception, it is not something that can be accurately and consistently gauged through tests or scans. The only way to verify the existence and intensity of pain is through truth and trust.

That means the reality of pain hinges on the sufferer's ability to convince others of its existence. I'll say that again. The sufferer must prove pain for its legitimacy to be accepted. *To have pain is to have certainty*, Elaine Scarry writes. *To hear about pain is to have doubt.* That means the sufferer must possess and be able to communicate the precise words, the correct scale, the accurate metaphors, the veiled cultural and contextual nuance, the courage, the humility, and the conviction of her pain. And, as if that were not enough, even if she manages to convey all these parts perfectly, the onus is on others (physicians, clinicians, family members, coworkers) to trust, to fully believe the sufferer when she claims her pain as real. Her experience must fit within the boundaries of culturally accepted versions of pain. She must fit the culturally accepted version of someone who is accepted to have pain. It helps when she has money. It helps when she is white. It helps when her sex is the same as her gender.

When was the last time you had to prove your pain?

Arrange the pieces that come your way.

I try to will myself well. I also try intravenous medication. Weekly yoga classes in bright, well-lit rooms with calming music and kind teachers. Vitamins and herbal mixtures and teas. Creams I massage into my neck. Anti-seizure medication. Hypnosis. Therapy. I even try doing nothing at all, longing for my body to correct itself naturally. I optimistically approach each new appointment with the hope it will be the one that offers relief. The important word here is *try*. Surely, this too, as everyone keeps saying, shall pass.

Still, I begin every morning in pain. I eat lunch in pain. I read books I mow the grass I deposit money in the bank I vote I hum I fuck I run until my feet ache and my legs burn: pain. In the wake of disturbance, I have concocted out of my days something that resembles life but is little more than well-placed debris.

I try medication with the side effect of eliminating any trace of hunger. Another makes my cheeks full and my stomach tight against the waistline of my jeans. One can only be used absent alcohol in my system. Another requires that I sit weekly in a beige outpatient room in the neurology department while an IV drips medication into my veins.

The mornings when my pain is silent, I work on an organic farm thinning beets, harvesting leeks, planting then labeling pallets of heirloom tomato starters. I pull ticks from my body. I use the nail of one finger to dislodge dirt caked under another. I tighten my belt. The farmer, hair the color of flames and a spirit to match, calls in the evening when the day's work is finally complete. He wants to know if he can bring dinner. Lettuce crisp, bright green and purple, potatoes warm with tarragon and oil. Delicate salmon, cool and pink. I taste lemon and mint, flakes of salt, the yellow wax beans still firm.

Potential Sources: An Inventory

List the foods you eat. Now stop eating those foods. It may be hormones responding to the indefatigable pull of the moon. If we look, will we find tumors on her spine, her brain, in her glands? Stress. Could she just be imagining the pain? We have a word for this. Women have been known. It must not be as bad as she says it is. She doesn't look like she's in pain. Or is there trauma hidden deep in her consciousness? Let's sit in this ripe moment as long as it takes. My next client won't be here for hours, tell me more about when you were a child, are you sure you were safe? Ask your body what is tunneling its way out the side of your head, is it her eyes or jaw or spinal alignment, those veiled hereditary traits from generations long buried in the dusty earth? Does it have a name? Is it a god? What about MS? Has anyone checked her chakras test her blood her urine are her thyroid levels normal? Let's try sedation.

Clinical Documentation

I spent thirty minutes today discussing further management of her headache. I have encouraged her to pursue MRI and the lumbar puncture. She apparently had a bad experience with the previous lumbar puncture in Colorado. I recommended that she ask for permission to take a small amount of Alprazolam prior to the test and that she be accompanied. In terms of her insomnia, I recommended that she go back to work and start exercising. She may take an occasional Alprazolam, less than one a week, and that I would refill that periodically if needed. In addition, she is going to the Mayo Clinic. I will be seeing her March 4 for a complete physical. We can follow up at that time. I recommended some books regarding mindfulness and recommended that she pursue the counseling as they have recommended. We also discussed side effects of the Topamax, increasing the dose slowly, and also discussed pregnancy problems with Topamax and did some pre-conceptual counseling. She is on birth control until we discuss this further and switch her meds but not for the next six months or so.

Absent a diagnosis, my time is spent worrying. I don't like this but we don't always get to choose what captures our attention. Remember: never underestimate the importance of control. The unknown elicits fear by projecting worst-case scenarios onto life's blank spaces. When left unresolved, fear has an unsightly way of morphing into anger. Which is better to say: I am worried or I hate this?

Remember: familiarity inspires in us a sense of control.

If I cannot escape it then I will do what I always do when faced with the unknown: I will attempt to learn this pain. I can control what I know.

I go online and search *headaches* then *headaches everyday* then *what causes headaches* then *headache that won't go away with medication* then *headache on both sides of your head above your ears and across your forehead* then *how to know when to go to the hospital for headache pain* then *natural pain relief for headaches* then *sharp pain behind one eye* then *what else can headache pain mean* then *how long can a headache last* then *other things that cause headaches* then *headaches in women* then *headaches in young healthy women* then *can headaches kill you* then *is it okay to drink if you have a headache* then *headache pain clinics* then *how to get a referral for headache pain clinics* then *foods to eat or avoid if you have a headache*.

On WebMD Symptom Checker, I enter my age and gender. The outline of a female body appears on my screen and I select the box indicating *headache*. I refine the search when asked to describe the headache. I choose: *pounding, dull, severe, headache in back of head, headache behind ears*. I roll my cursor over the body to indicate soreness in the neck. Before it displays my results, WebMD asks if I could be pregnant. The conditions that match my symptoms are *Migraine Headache, Cluster Headache, Cerebellar Hemorrhage, Tension Headache, Acute Sinusitis, Pneumococcal Meningitis, Influenza, Whiplash, Meningitis, Cervical Spondylosis*.

Searching the internet for answers is like walking through a house of warped mirrors. The accredited sites are weighed down by cumbersome statistics and sterile case studies. They offer information but fail to satisfy my hunger for understanding. Blog posts about how to deal with headache pain inevitably recommend meditation. Forum posts by well-intentioned but ultimately hopeless sufferers spiral endlessly. The worst-case scenarios—hemorrhages, tumors, cancers—filter to the top of every search list.

The internet solves many problems, but unidentified pain is not one of them. Each time I try to engage the wider world for answers, I end up walking away from the computer discouraged to my core, overwhelmed by the depth of unsolved hurt that lingers online, frustrated that the questions I ask fail to result in succinct answers. I long for the revelation I hoped an expanded community would provide. But the scattered information and the contradictory voices are dizzying, not settling. I feel more alone than ever.

The internet inspires fear more than certainty, so it becomes anathema. I make a deliberate choice to not engage health-related queries online.

Instead, I read books. I read one suggesting pain is like the magnetic needle inside a compass. The needle's primary objective is to guide the explorer in the correct direction, a direction that leads ultimately to the source—the illness, the injury—responsible for the pain. Fair enough. But who am I in this metaphor? The compass? The destination? The trampled ground below the explorer's blistered feet? The sun low on the horizon? I appear to be all the parts all at once. Pain is the needle, that much I know. That means I am somehow both the problem and the solution. (Paradox.) To complicate the matter, the needle in my internal compass appears to be broken. It spins inside the confines of the compass, irreverent, erratic, without purpose or aim, indifferent to the pull of the magnetic true north. Without a true north I am directionless.

Directionless but not idle.

The needle always points to something.

So I wander the path where the needle points searching for a source, or at the very least, the suggestion of a source. Along the way, I am learning all sorts of things. I learn it's best to wear glasses, not contacts, when pain knots itself deep into my temples. I learn not to tuck my chin to my chest when I sleep. I learn a lot about what helps other people when they have headaches. *Yes, I tried yoga. Really, vitamin B did all that for you? My next appointment is Wednesday. No, but thank you, I'll borrow a copy from the library.*

But even the knowledge gained from wandering does not lead to the source. There has been no injury, virus, or weakening. I do not appear to have a syndrome. What I have is pain that won't go away. What complicates the matter is that at times the struggle isn't even the pain itself but rather everything that surrounds it: the appointments that require a steady renewal of physical and emotional vulnerability, the constant explanations, the guessing, the attempts at renewed hope. The worrying. The waiting rooms. My god, the waiting rooms. The bills, the co-payments, the phone calls with the insurance agents. How pain filters into every conversation, every decision. Doctors tell me again and again and again: pain is not a diagnosis, it is a symptom. The neurologist, a tall man in his sixties with a gray beard who looks as though he has slept in his clothes, says to me, *I know you want answers, but you don't want them to come from me.*

To Whom It May Concern,

was in   distress

it was

normal

normal.   normal
normal.
normal

normal

normal.

Clinical Documentation

FINAL REPORT

Examination: Brain MRI, without contrast

Indication: Headaches

Procedure: Multiplanar T1, T2, FLAIR, and gradient T2 acquisitions obtained

Findings: Ventricular size and contour are normal, no midline shift. Gray-white matter interface normal. Prominent perivascular markings of bilateral basal ganglia anteriorly. Midbrain, hindbrain, and cerebellar hemispheres are normal. No bright signal white matter foci seen. Anterior and posterior circulation patent. Sinuses are normal. Orbits unremarkable. Normal CP angles. Cervicomedullary junction and pituitary gland are normal. No blood products.

It's true, I do want answers. Because without them, something else inevitably fills the void where answers should be. It's difficult to ascribe meaning to the unknown when it feels like I don't even have a proper vocabulary from which to choose.

It's difficult to speak about pain without also speaking about fear. Fear is worry's worry. It is the ultimate void-filler. It's opportunistic. Like an infection, it worms its way into compromised bodies, attaching eagerly to each shiny, wet surface where it breeds irresponsibly. Fear embeds itself in bones, into stiff muscles, alongside worn tendons. Broken bodies are a perfect host.

I'm not afraid of dying. As best as I can I have made peace with my own mortality. Death is a fixed consequence of life, an event uncompromising to the most potent of arguments and persuasions. And yet for some reason I fear dying from this strange, incurable, untraceable malfunction that is trapped inside my body. I don't want this to be the thing that kills me. Maybe it's just another grasp at control. Or maybe this is what it looks like to fight for your life.

I am afraid of this pain.

You would be, too.

When the pain shifts, when it bursts sharp across my forehead, or when it pulls unevenly behind my eyes, I am afraid it will consume my entire body. When I wake in the middle of the night because the beat of my pulse is heavy in my temples, or my neck is aching and stiff, I am afraid I will never feel well again. Making plans feels like a gamble because the pain is so unpredictable. Not knowing how I will feel in the future makes commitment a fearful thing. Will the foods I eat, the shoes I wear, the bed I sleep in, the medicine I consume, the banal activities of my day make the pain worse? How much worse? What's my breaking point? How much pain can I handle? How will I know my own limits? I am afraid the pain will never end. I am afraid of what will happen when it expands beyond what feels normal or what I am able to handle. I am afraid of what I might be forced to do to quiet the noise. I am afraid something—a blood vessel, a clotted vein, an unseen tumor, my soul— will erupt. I am afraid the pain will alter my life in irreversible ways. I am afraid of what it means to live in a constant state of unknowing. I fear this pain will remain nameless, a glitch in an otherwise functioning system. My logic chases its own tail: a name means a cure and a cure means I won't always feel this way. But if the pain remains nameless, causeless, and cureless, then I guess it really isn't even a problem at all. The pain is just me. I am a person in a broken body. I am the pain. The pain is me. How do you classify the nameless? What do you call pain without beginning or end? The word *purgatory* comes to mind.

Pain: A Primer

Pain is an unpleasant sensory and emotional experience associated with, or resembling that associated with, actual or potential tissue damage. Pain is always a personal experience that is influenced to varying degrees by biological, psychological, and social factors. Pain and nociception are different phenomena. Pain cannot be inferred solely from activity in sensory neurons. Through their life experiences, individuals learn the concept of pain. A person's report of an experience as pain should be respected. Although pain usually serves an adaptive role, it may have adverse effects on function and social and psychological well-being. Verbal description is only one of several behaviors to express pain; inability to communicate does not negate the possibility that a human or a nonhuman animal experiences pain.

Vocabulary Lessons

_____:

(verb) I want a word for the internal stillness triggered by pain.

You will want to take your time when you say it out loud. There is a complication in the middle that requires careful enunciation. The word is uneven when you write it on a page but don't let that dissuade you from using it. There are more letters involved than you may think necessary. It's mostly vowels. It's easy to misspell. You can't take it back. When you say it in an empty room, it may feel like you are purring.

Used in a sentence:

On the couch, head to pillow, feet under the blanket, fire across the room, mesmerized by _____.

Classifications

Black holes. The dark matter of the brain. Infinity. Zero. We name the unknown so that we might someday understand it. This is how we make sense of the unfamiliar. It's how we dignify experience. How we recategorize the unknown into the familiar. It's storytelling. It's metaphor. It's how we distill corporate realities into specific, personal experiences: we create minor categories of major undertakings.

Heliotrope. Nymphea. Archil.

Mathematician Alexander Grothendieck believed that naming afforded cognitive power over that which is yet to be understood. He would, it was noted, choose *striking and evocative names for new concepts* because he believed the very act of naming unknown, not-yet understood concepts was a necessary part of the process of discovery. Once named, these unruly concepts could be handled, understood, and then, ultimately, controlled.

Livid. Sepia. Fallow.

We name the pigments that create our world. There is a color named after an Italian racecar that trekked from Peking to Paris (Rosso Corsa). There is one named after a curious botanist (Fuchsia). We named marine ooze (Chalk). We named grief (Cerulean). We named status (Tyrian Purple). These pigments tell the story of history, the history of art.

Some are named for herbal concoctions (Absinthe), some are old (Umber), others new (Fluorescent Pink).

Carl Linnaeus, an eighteenth-century Swedish botanist, zoologist, and physician, developed a system for classifying the animal kingdom that is still used today. Linnaeus used consistent language to identify and classify animal life based on shared physical characteristics, a practice now known as taxonomy. The seven levels of animal classification according to Linnaeus are kingdom, phylum, class, order, family, genus, and species.

Naples Yellow. Citrine.

We categorize the functions and structures of the body into interdependent systems so that we can better recognize how the whole is greater than the sum of its parts. Circulation, Digestion, Endocrine. Muscle. Immune and Integumentary. Nervous. Renal, Respiratory, and Reproductive. Skeletal and Hematopoietic.

Dutch Orange.

Words belong to each other.

Clinical Documentation

Examination: MRA of the circle of Willis

Indication: Headaches

Procedure: Axial plane time of flight was obtained with MIP imaging in both horizontal and vertical rotations.

Findings: Anterior circulation from carotid canal superiorly through siphon into A1 and P1 segments demonstrates normal caliber vessels, no obvious intraluminal pathology. Anterior communicating vessel is not well delineated. No evidence of posterior communicating arteries. No vessel irregular nor aneurysms present. Basilar vertebral vessel is normal. P1 segments normal. Superior cerebellar branch is ill-defined. Posterior communicating vessels are absent, a developmental variant.

How much pain can you handle?

The room is not small, though it feels that way.

Books and papers tower every surface, giving the impression of a crowded cityscape. I struggle to focus with such disorder vying for my attention. Desperate for relief from what has become an all-consuming, yearslong headache, I cross state lines for an appointment at the Mayo Clinic in Rochester, Minnesota. The doctor, unfazed by the chaos closing in on us, speaks; the staccato rhythm of pen on paper records my attempts at answers. His hair grays at the temples. He slouches over his desk in the manner of a man more comfortable with books than with people. It looks as though he forgot to shave.

He does not meet my eyes.

This headache that will not go away is like an alarm that sounds though there is no longer a fire.

Speak illness as metaphor and I will understand.

Speak illness as metaphor and metaphor it will indelibly remain.

There is no fire. There is no smoke. Our job is to figure out how to remove the batteries.

Medical Metaphor: A Primer

Physicians use metaphor to create a common language with their patients. Borrowing known symbols and figures of speech allows physicians to communicate unknown and often complex medical explanations. This practice proves a helpful tool for both patients and physicians working to connote cultural assumptions and attitudes. Common illness metaphors are as follows.

Illness is an enemy attacker. Infected cells invade healthy tissue. Wounds are vulnerable to infection. Your body fights off illness. Medications work to strengthen your body's defenses. We must fight off illness like an attacker. We must resist infection. *Illness is a war.* The body does battle, engages in struggles, fights the good fight. We either beat illness or we succumb. You are given the all clear. There are outbreaks, flare-ups, bouts, fits—as in conflicts. *Illness is an unnatural state.* Those who are ill become shadows or ghosts of their former selves. You are out of sorts. You are a victim. *Illness is monochrome.* The sick are described as white, ashen, gray, green. Your color is off. You fade away.

On the metaphorical plane, illness is lower than health. You fall ill or come down with a sickness. You are laid low. You collapse or keel over. Illness can strike us down. We feel low, run-down, under the weather. We are sinking fast. Or, when connoting health, one might bounce back. We get back on our feet. You are on the up-and-up.

The metaphors we use—whether medical, religious, or otherwise—matter because our lexical choices define us. They suggest shape and structure requisite to identity. The

words we use concentrate the mind by asserting productive narratives, both to ourselves and to the world at large,
of that which is true. Metaphors allow room to authenticate
the nameless. They provide a script outlining behavior and
expectations. They challenge loneliness. What I am trying
to say is that when we give something a name, we give it
an identity.

My pain remains nameless.

I think of the Egyptian deity Ptah who possessed the power to create anything that he could first name. I think of the miller's daughter who claimed agency over her fate only after she learned the name of the imp Rumpelstiltskin. I think of how Adam was given the responsibility of naming cattle, naming birds, naming each paraded animal. In these stories, these metaphors of power and domination, we transform the mysterious into the known.

If doctors can't and won't, what name will I give this pain?

I ignored my initial instinct that this doctor would not be a good fit.

Her desk was comical. What I mean is that it was covered with stuffed animals and cheap glass trinkets of animated film characters, as though she believed the invocation of innocence had the power to ease pain.

What does the pain feel like? She condescends.

The question is wrong; therefore, my answer is wrong.

It feels like pain, I respond.

Well, duh, she retorts.

What does it feel like? It feels like my brain has been replaced by a heavy stone. It feels like a convex metal bar pressing a concave hollow into the side of my head. My blood feels like basalt. It feels like my eyes are cramping from dehydration. It feels like my cheekbones are bruised. It feels like untouchable sonic uproar resonates in each ear. My forehead feels as though it is splintering apart like dry wood tossed on a roaring fire. My muscles feel like ropes wrenched in opposite directions. Like my veins are on the wrong side of my skin, like a tourniquet of concertina wire prevents blood from leaving my skull. It feels like a worm eating the words out of my mouth. It feels like a prism of light caught in my eye. It feels like each vertebra in my spine is a weight pulling my head to the ground. It feels like an infected wound that never heals. It feels like an engine running at full speed in the wrong gear. Like I am on the wrong side of the door. Like everything I do, no matter how hard I try, is wrong. I never knew I could be this many forms of wrong. It feels like a sliver of glass on a bare foot. Like I am holding a dead bird in my hands. What does it feel like? It feels like punishment, like regret, like the thief of hope, like the hem of the cloak trailing behind Charon as he walks briskly to the underworld.

Is that the answer you are looking for?

Classifications

Gray. Gainsboro. Silver. Slate and Metallic. Spanish or Davy's. Jet and Xanadu. Platinum, Ash, Gunmetal. Battleship. Nickel. Stone, Cadet. Glaucous. Marengo and Payne. Puce and Cinereous. French.

A watch of nightingales. A huddle of penguins. A muster of storks. An aerie of eagles. A cote of doves. A raft of ducks. A tiding of magpies. An unkindness of ravens.

Migraines. Tension headaches. Cluster headaches.

Vocabulary Lessons

Patient:

(adjective and noun) Enduring pain, affliction, inconvenience, etc., calmly, without discontent or complaint; characterized by or showing such endurance. Able to wait calmly; quietly expectant; not hasty or impetuous. Forbearing, long-suffering; tolerant of the faults or limitations of other people. A sufferer, especially one who endures suffering without complaint. Of multiple origins. Partly a borrowing from French. Partly a borrowing from Latin. Derived from the same Indo-European base as the ancient Greek πῆμα, meaning "suffering."

Used in a sentence:

My nature to be a patient patient both serves me well and undercuts the care I receive.

With each movement the paper below my thighs crinkles loudly. Instinctually, the palm of my hand works to smooth the wrinkles flat against the tan vinyl examination table. It feels as though I have been here before. This is a copy of every examination room in every doctor's office in every city.

On the back of the door is an anatomy chart outlining the categorized systems of a toned male body, a flawless specimen of health. Why do these charts only ever depict male bodies? Am I to assume that female bodies are interchangeable with the male bodies save for their respective reproductive functions? Are females just smaller versions of males?

My nature is to be a patient patient. To sit, back straight, quiet, to smile, to say yes. To wait as long as it takes. To abide by the guiding moral principle that problems have solutions. To fall into the expected line of authority. To assume that, unlike me, doctors have access to said solutions. These cultural expectations are embedded in my character, difficult to dismiss. I have no reason to believe otherwise.

And yet, I am beginning to wonder if maybe I should believe otherwise.

One hour and twenty minutes in the windowless office pass before he enters the room. He does not shake my hand. He does not introduce himself. I swallow hard and look at his face. His features are more suited for a young boy than a grown man, a genetic shortcoming for which he compensates with palpable arrogance. Had I bowed or made a motion to kiss his hand, I imagine he would not have been surprised.

He eyes my chart suspiciously.

What brings you in today? It says here you have a headache.

Hypothesized Internal Monologue
of Said Late Physician

Anonymous girl with headaches she's probably pregnant or just stressed that she's not yet pregnant did the nurse do a pregnancy test isn't today the day the hot pharmaceutical rep brings lunch Christ I hope it's not Panera again remember to tell her to sign out when she leaves the nurse at the front will need her insurance card and co-pay fuck it's only ten thirty

Vocabulary Lessons

Hysteria:

(noun) A physical disorder of women attributed to displacement or dysfunction of the uterus and characterized by neurological symptoms often accompanied by exaggeratedly or inappropriately emotional behavior, originally attributed to disease or injury of the nervous system and later thought to be functional or psychogenic in origin. A borrowing from the Latin *hysterica*, meaning "of the womb."

Used in a sentence:

He knows he can't and knows he shouldn't and knows it won't even be an accurate diagnosis if he does, but still, he wants to tell me what I have is nothing more than a bout of hysteria.

Hysteria: A Primer

Even when it shouldn't, it always comes back to the uterus.

The definition, diagnosis, and treatment for hysteria, a disease historically and predominantly attributed to women, is unknown, contested, and often misunderstood. Some believe the first depictions of the unruly physical and emotional disturbance date back as far as 1900 BC, but because of its etymology most attribute the discovery of illness to the Greeks.

One theory is that Hippocrates, the so-called father of medicine who lived in Greece around the fifth century BC, *freed the emerging science from the chains of superstition, introduced empirical observation and the bedside manner, and both identified and named "hysteria."* Hippocrates initiated the belief that disease originated within the body and was not, as had been previously believed, sanctioned by the gods. He went on to parse the differences between the male and female bodies, which is how he arrived at the conclusion that *the womb is the origin of all diseases.*

Centuries later, Greek physicians posited that illness was a systemic process, meaning that it occurred within and throughout the entire mind, body, and soul. In their view, no distinction was to be made between the body and the mind. It was their job as physicians to identify and thereby reestablish the equilibrium that had been distorted in their patients' bodies. Around the second century, Aretaeus, a Cappadocian physician, posited the ailments that afflicted women were a result of the uterus, which was susceptible to detachment and could float throughout the body.

Once the wandering uterus landed, it was believed to put inordinate pressure on other organs, thereby causing the presenting symptoms and discomforts. Aretaeus believed that while in motion, the wandering womb traveled the body in search of fluids, moving toward pleasing smells and away from fetid ones, roving inside the body like *an animal within the animal*. Soranus, also a Greek physician, likened the uterus not to a tamed animal but to a wild beast.

The idea that hysteria was the result of a wandering womb was rejected by Aretaeus's contemporary Galen. Instead, the Roman physician argued that the unnatural or troubling symptoms that were exhibited primarily in women—anxiety, fainting, sexual desire, insomnia, irritability, loss of appetite for food, or, ironically, loss of appetite for sex—were the result of retained substances within the uterus, specifically female semen and menstrual blood. Treatment of the condition known as hysteria or hysterical suffocation was administered by fumigation, suppositories of burnt sulfur and asphalt in honey, wine, smoke from an extinguished lamp wick, and, some believe, by regular climax or sexual intercourse with a spouse. Marriage or pregnancy were deemed the most effective treatments. For those without a husband, doctors and midwives were suitable substitutes for helping patients reach orgasm, a treatment called hysterical paroxysm, although masturbation by the inflicted woman was not a recommended course of treatment.

The theory of the wandering womb persisted until the Middle Ages, when demonic possession, witchcraft, and melancholy grew in popularity as the go-to diagnoses for troublesome women and the bodies they occupied.

Around the 1680s, a pair of English physicians advanced the medicalization of hysteria and its place in society. Thomas Sydenham put forth two observations that altered how hysteria was diagnosed and perceived. First, though most cases were diagnosed in women, Sydenham believed that men were also susceptible to hysteria. Second, Sydenham claimed that hysteria did not originate in the uterus but was instead a *disease of civilization*. The implication of Sydenham's belief was that the demands of society, most notably those felt by the rich and those with delicate nerves, increased susceptibility to the disease.

Sydenham's contemporary, Thomas Willis, agreed that hysteria affected both men and women, though he maintained, somehow, that the condition was rooted in the uterus. Anatomical oversight aside, Willis contributed to the classification of hysteria by designating the disease a disorder of the nervous system. Though men and women possessed the same symptomatic issues, men were often diagnosed with melancholy, whereas women were diagnosed with hysteria.

In the eighteenth century, on account of advances made because of medical and scientific discovery, the classification of hysteria was fully embraced as a disorder not of the uterus but of the brain—specifically, as Willis had previously claimed, a disease of the nervous system. It was a designation that legitimized the illness and, for a time, contributed to its appeal by ushering it under the wing of medicine practiced by respected physicians and away from the *ill-defined conditions such as the vapors, melancholy, and hypochondria.*

Throughout the nineteenth century, physicians narrowed the definition of illness by using scientific and medical advances to link presenting symptoms with specific malfunctions of the body. Medical specialties such as gynecology and neurology came into favor *in no small part because of their claims to own the treatment for hysteria.* Asylums were established to accommodate the influx of patients diagnosed with the newly minted neurological diseases, and *while madness or lunacy wasn't yet gendered as a diagnosis, often the only difference between women diagnosed as mad and those diagnosed as hysterics was their wealth.* Rest cures, along with changes in diet and exercise, were commonly advised for affected patients.

The century came to a close with Jean-Martin Charcot, a French physician, who boldly theorized that hysteria was the result of a *sexually diseased and morally debauched female imagination.* Charcot, whose theories were studied and expounded upon by Sigmund Freud, maintained that hysteria was a gendered disease that affected women and was curable by hypnosis. Freud posited that hysteria was the result of childhood sexual abuse, a theory he maintained until, ravaged by grief after the death of his own father, he himself experienced similar symptoms.

By the late twentieth century, in response to advancements that correctly explained how some of the disorders previously attributed to hysteria were better classified elsewhere, the American Psychological Association altered the definition of hysteria from hysterical neurosis, conversion type—a diagnosis that attributed the disease not to neurological deficits but instead to psychogenic stress and emotional conflicts—to conversion disorder—a condition in which a person experiences physical and sensory problems absent any underlying neurological pathology. This reclassification led to a steady decline in reported diagnosis of the disease. In response to this decline, hysteria was removed from the *Diagnostic and Statistical Manual of Mental Disorders* in 1980.

Though the name, definition, diagnosis, and treatment of hysteria has evolved and mutated over time, what remains consistent is that hysteria has been a catch-all for the unidentifiable ailments found in a complaining woman's body.

Headaches, for example.

Who knows? Maybe I am hysterical.

I forget things. Sometimes my emotions run surface deep. Other times they are a threatening whirlwind, a hazard to anyone who dares come close to the disaster that is my life. I am stressed. I do wear this stress on my body like a heavy garment. I wouldn't mind some attention.

I do have a uterus.

But does the suffering originate from my womb? Is there an animal within me, clawing her way to the surface? If you turned me inside out, would we find evidence of her being? Would there be marks scratched into my belly where she dragged her claws? Is it a womb or a den? *What does the pain feel like?* What does suffering feel like? Because I don't think they are the same thing at all, but I do picture the two holding hands. Is suffering encompassing like rage? Or is it utterly silent, callous, or maybe even slightly anxious? Does suffering feel like endurance? If pain is the journey of the body, is suffering the journey of the soul? That sounds like something they want me to believe is true.

Suffering. Is that why this evening with friends feels like I am wearing clothes that don't fit? Why I lost my energy today? Or was that the pain? Is that why it feels like I have lost control over my life? Why I yelled at you? My life is deteriorating. My body is deteriorating. Wouldn't you be angry, too? Because the pain won't quit. It just won't quit and no one seems to know why. It's elusive like a shadow. Like quiet. Like God. Like coming. Like the last lick of smoke evaporating into the night air as embers pulse their dying heat.

It could be anything, so why not an animal, why not a beast, why not this?

Risk Factors

MEDICATION RISK FACTORS

Medicine can slow or stop your breathing and death may occur.

Long-term use may affect fertility.

Can sometimes cause personality changes that affect the way you behave, react, feel, or interact with others.

May cause agitation, aggression, or other behavior problems.

May cause mood changes, such as anxiety, mood swings, and depression.

Medication may raise your risk for suicidal thoughts or behaviors.

May cause dizziness, confusion, mood swings, headache, tiredness, diarrhea, sleep changes, and brief feelings similar to electric shock.

Hives, difficulty breathing, swelling of your lips, tongue, face, or throat.

Painful urination.

Twitching or loss of coordination.

Seeing things that aren't there (hallucinations).

Nightmares.

Perhaps

I think of all the women, centuries upon centuries of women, who lived their lives in actual real pain. Women brave or broken enough to seek answers, women with nothing left to give, women with everything left to give, women with resources, women with none; the aching, the brittle, the fevered, the breathless, the cautious; women who demanded answers, women unable to respond, unable to talk back, unable to say no, unable to ask; mothers, daughters, grandmothers, a woman on her own, someone's sister, someone's chosen; women who were not believed, women who were mocked, women who were told they were imagining, women who were told they were crazy, women who were told they couldn't possibly, women who were told they were seeking attention, who were told they just needed to rest, women who were told they were whores; the hopeless, the penniless, the unhoused, the vulnerable; women who were lied to, women who were abused by their physicians, women who were given unauthorized treatments, women who were experimented on, women who were given aspirin; women who suffered alone, women who cried in the night, women who had their children taken from them, women who had their wombs taken from them, women who had their careers taken from them, women who had portions of their brains taken from them; those who were tired, those whose bodies would not let them relax, those who hid their pain from everyone, those who spoke their truth aloud for everyone to hear, those who wouldn't be quiet; the women who would rather die than keep living, the women who killed themselves, the women who lived their entire lives in pain; the women caught in-between.

I may be a paradox, but history proves I am not an anomaly.

Sex Differences: A Primer

Male-unless-otherwise-indicated has been the default slant, a secondary position designated to females that has influenced the understanding of sex differences throughout the ages. Anatomically, the Greeks believed ovaries were the female's version of testicles and that the uterus was the equivalent of a scrotum. The female, or as she was described, the male *turned outside in*, was more or less seen as a mutation, the tragic result of a biological deficiency in *vital heat*. Aristotle, thinking this to be true, characterized the female body as *a mutilated male.*

Is this centuries-old misogyny why the distinction was made between anatomy and female anatomy? Or why the focus on women's health so often centers exclusively on reproduction?

Researchers have identified sex differences in every tissue and organ system in the human body, as well as in *the prevalence, course and severity of the majority of common human diseases*. In full awareness of this conclusion, the practice of researching predominately male bodies then applying said findings to female bodies continues. It is not uncommon for the results from clinical trials to be presented as valid for males and females even when females have been excluded from studies.

The United States Food and Drug Administration (FDA) states that the second most common adverse drug reaction in female bodies is simply that the drug in question doesn't work, even though the same drug was proven to work in male bodies. Though females consume approximately

80 percent of pharmaceuticals in the United States, these same people are often excluded from clinical trials to test drugs because of their *fluctuating, "atypical" hormones*, which have been known to affect the efficacy of the drugs in question. This result begs the question: How many drugs that could possibly work for females have been ruled out during phase one trials because they had no effect on the males on which they were exclusively tested? Do researchers not know what causes pain in the female body because medicine is a gendered institution where 70 percent of chronic pain patients are females but 80 percent of pain studies are conducted on men or male mice?

In 1993, the FDA and the National Institutes of Health (NIH) mandated the inclusion of women in clinical trials. This decision reversed a decades-old policy that excluded females of childbearing potential from early-stage drug trials. The initial reason given for this dramatic exclusion was that since females are born with all the eggs their bodies will ever produce, for their safety and the safety of their unborn children, they should not be exposed to any potential hazardous toxins that may hinder their reproductive abilities. This mandate declared that all females, no matter their age, gender status, sexual orientation, or wish or ability to bear children, were excluded from clinical drug trials.

Though the mandate has been reversed, it continues to be the case that trial results are not always analyzed for sex differences. Females continue to be excluded from clinical and preclinical trials because, according to some researchers, the unpredictable nature of their hormones introduces too much variability.

Only since 2016 has the NIH ruled that pain drugs must be tested in female rodents as well as males. Even though chronic pain affects as many people as the combination of cancer, heart disease, and diabetes, it still receives 95 percent less funding. Why is that the case? Why have we continued to let that be the case? Is this because chronic pain disrupts but doesn't actually kill those affected? Or is it because the majority of those whose lives it disrupts are female, not male? Where do we draw the line on lives worth saving? If pain affected as many males as it does females, would the urgency to solve the problem of pain be heightened? Because right now there is no equivalent: there is not a single destructive but nonfatal disease that affects twice as many males as females.

My primary care physician recommends I make an appointment with a therapist, *you know,* she says, raising her shoulder in the suggestion of a shrug, *to talk through how all of this is affecting your life.*

Clinical Documentation

Headaches, unclear etiology. Patient has had extensive workups over the past year, none of which have helped whatsoever. No etiologies have been found. Because she did score mild-to-moderate depression on her Beck's Depression Inventory, we will start her on Cymbalta daily. We discussed benefits and risks as well as side effects of the medication, and we will see her again in three weeks. In the meanwhile, I think it is reasonable to obtain a new set of screening labs, and therefore, will beta a CBC, urine dip, CMP, lead, sed rate, CRP, and a heavy-metal screen.

a   woman who denies

            evaluation   her doctor's
                                . She

            was clearly

    She denies   aggravated
                                          change

                                                    she lies

She cannot think
                                    She is

                                              without significant
                                    benefit.

96

Data Collection: Beck Depression Inventory

The Beck Depression Inventory was created by psychiatrist Aaron Beck in 1961. Beck, an influential physician and the pioneer of cognitive therapy and cognitive behavioral therapy, created the twenty-one-question, multiple-choice, self-reported inventory to be used as a psychometric test for measuring the severity of depression. The purpose of the inventory is to detect, assess, and monitor changes patients exhibit regarding depressive symptoms.

Data Collection: Beck Depression Inventory

1. 0 I do not feel sad.
   1 I feel sad.
   2 I am sad all the time and I can't snap out of it.
   3 I am so sad and unhappy that I can't stand it.

2. 0 I am not particularly discouraged about the future.
   1 I feel discouraged about the future.
   2 I feel I have nothing to look forward to.
   3 I feel the future is hopeless and that things cannot improve.

3. 0 I do not feel like a failure.
   1 I feel I have failed more than the average person.
   2 As I look back on my life, all I can see is a lot of failures.
   3 I feel I am a complete failure as a person.

4. 0 I get as much satisfaction out of things as I used to.
   1 I don't enjoy things the way I used to.
   2 I don't get real satisfaction out of anything anymore.
   3 I am dissatisfied or bored with everything.

5. 0 I don't feel particularly guilty.
   1 I feel guilty a good part of the time.
   2 I feel quite guilty most of the time.
   3 I feel guilty all of the time.

6. 0 I don't feel I am being punished.
   1 I feel I may be punished.
   2 I expect to be punished.
   3 I feel I am being punished.

7. 0 I don't feel disappointed in myself.
   1 I am disappointed in myself.
   2 I am disgusted with myself.
   3 I hate myself.

8. 0 I don't feel I am any worse than anybody else.
   1 I am critical of myself for my weaknesses or mistakes.
   2 I blame myself all the time for my faults.
   3 I blame myself for everything bad that happens.

9. 0 I don't have any thoughts of killing myself.
   1 I have thoughts of killing myself, but I would not carry them out.
   2 I would like to kill myself.
   3 I would kill myself if I had the chance.

10. 0 I don't cry any more than usual.
    1 I cry more now than I used to.
    2 I cry all the time now.
    3 I used to be able to cry, but now I can't cry even though I want to.

11. 0 I am no more irritated by things than I ever was.
    1 I am slightly more irritated now than usual.
    2 I am quite annoyed or irritated a good deal of the time.
    3 I feel irritated all the time.

12. 0 I have not lost interest in other people.
    1 I am less interested in other people than I used to be.
    2 I have lost most of my interest in other people.
    3 I have lost all of my interest in other people.

13. 0 I make decisions about as well as I ever could.
    1 I put off making decisions more than I used to.
    2 I have greater difficulty in making decisions more than I used to.
    3 I can't make decisions at all anymore.

14. 0 I don't feel that I look any worse than I used to.
    1 I am worried that I am looking old or unattractive.
    2 I feel there are permanent changes in my appearance that make me look unattractive.
    3 I believe that I look ugly.

15. 0 I can work about as well as before.
    1 It takes an extra effort to get started at doing something.
    2 I have to push myself very hard to do anything.
    3 I can't do any work at all.

16. 0 I can sleep as well as usual.
    1 I don't sleep as well as I used to.
    2 I wake up 1–2 hours earlier than usual and find it hard to get back to sleep.
    3 I wake up several hours earlier than I used to and cannot get back to sleep.

17. 0 I don't get more tired than usual.
    1 I get tired more easily than I used to.
    2 I get tired from doing almost anything.
    3 I am too tired to do anything.

18. 0 My appetite is no worse than usual.
    1 My appetite is not as good as it used to be.
    2 My appetite is much worse now.
    3 I have no appetite at all anymore.

19. 0 I haven't lost much weight, if any, lately.
    1 I have lost more than five pounds.
    2 I have lost more than ten pounds.
    3 I have lost more than fifteen pounds.

20. 0 I am no more worried about my health than usual.
    1 I am worried about physical problems like aches, pains, upset stomach, or constipation.
    2 I am very worried about physical problems and it's hard to think of much else.
    3 I am so worried about my physical problems that I cannot think of anything else.

21. 0 I have not noticed any recent change in my interest in sex.
    1 I am less interested in sex than I used to be.
    2 I have almost no interest in sex.
    3 I have lost interest in sex completely.

The irony of this thwarted attention is not lost on me. I live in a culture obsessed with judging, controlling, monitoring, shaming, hiding, exploiting, denying, claiming, but not actually healing, my body.

There's more than one way to contain an animal within an animal.

Two parallel lines appear almost instantly across the small oval window. For all that my body doesn't do, this, apparently, it does well. I smile then rest my forehead against the wall. Stillness buttresses the moment. My body has done what I asked it to do. Beautifully. Quickly. Without intervention or delay. I allow the unfamiliar sensation as much room as it needs to be fully felt. The possibility of change commands the room. It lasts forever. It lasts only a few seconds.

When I tell him, his reaction mirrors my own. He smiles then places the palms of both hands against his temples. We laugh.

My pregnancy is utterly unremarkable.

I sleep, consistently, deeply, for the first time since the pain began two years ago and wake each morning caught in the residual inertia of dreams. At the hospital for a routine prenatal exam, the sound of a rapid heartbeat fills the room. I am sitting cross-legged on an overstuffed chair when I feel the first flutter, like a butterfly flapping its wings, against the inside edge of my belly.

For the first time in years when I visit the doctor, I am not anxious. I step on the scale, let the nurse take my blood pressure. *These are good,* she assures me as she types the numbers into my online chart. She asks: *Any pain today?* I hesitate. *Not really. I mean, I have a headache, but I always have headaches and this one isn't too bad.* She hesitates as well, her eyes locked on the screen, her fingers poised above the keyboard ready to record. *But no pain that's related to the pregnancy?* she asks without taking her eyes off the screen. I am quick, and honest, in my answer. *No.*

The midwife stretches the tape across my swollen belly and tells me I am progressing nicely. My blood sugar levels are average. I welcome the normalcy of these appointments where each question I ask has a clear, known answer. My headaches are a footnote to a larger story, something that deserves attention but is not the major issue at hand.

I can lean into this new life because it is a story that makes sense. It has boundaries and language and examples and rules. If my body can do this, then maybe it can be healed.

Vocabulary Lessons

_____:

(verb) I want a word for the polite smile I offer when people suggest *maybe pregnancy will cure your headaches.*

The word likely has an ancient etymology. It rises from your hip bones, forcing a roll almost like a growl in the back of your throat when you speak it. The louder you say it, the truer it becomes. The word will catch you off guard. It will clash with all your furniture. It will leave a mark like a lash on your skin. Don't be surprised if it sucks all the air out of the room.

Used in a sentence:

She _____ because it is rude to say *fuck you* to a complete stranger.

I crave the quotidian.

With the life I had planned now otherwise dismantled, the ordinary assumes an attractive, attainable appeal. I'll tend the garden. I'll get to know my neighbors as I walk the block. I'll read books and learn to sew. I'll harvest the basil and freeze pesto for the winter. I'll fill my time with temperate activities that I genuinely enjoy so that when I am forced to step back from it all, on account of not feeling well, the consequences will be minimal.

This measured posture is tolerable with one exception. When I think about the time I am losing, when I compare it to the time and energy afforded to my peers, anxiety churns in my gut. I am overwhelmed by an urgency to catch up, to prove my viability. The thing is, I can't figure out how to move forward while still carrying the weight of this unresolved problem inside my body. It is as if I am trying to win some arbitrary award for holding the most still. I stand, alert but frozen, muscles trembling from exhaustion, feverishly hoping to be rewarded for my heroic solitary effort.

I am desperate to leave behind the uncertainty of the last few years, the unknowing and unpredictability of pain. I am tired of always think-ing about pain. I have grown fatigued trying to solve this frustrated riddle that has become my life. I don't want to talk about it anymore: not to him, not to my therapist, not to my friends. It's time for my body to produce something good, not just something damaged. Maybe for once I can fit in. Maybe I can leave the margin behind. Maybe if I do this one thing right then everything else will fall into place.

A body that gestates properly. A body that aches improperly.

Even as my body performs pregnancy perfectly, I am in near-constant pain. As if to follow suit, my thoughts split down the middle. Thinking this way becomes an obsessive pattern, a rut into which I fall daily, an oscillation between cause and cure, between health and dis-ease.

It looks like nesting but it's really an attempt to distract myself from the pain. I empty the refrigerator of its contents, wipe down each surface with a natural disinfectant, and throw away the half-empty bottles of condiments that take up space. I donate bags of unwanted clothes to the thrift store. At Target I purchase matching fabric bins and five-tiered wire shelving racks for the basement. The racks are heavier than what I should be carrying, but somehow I manage to maneuver the boxes down the stairs so I can assemble them piece by piece. I sit in a narrow rectangle of space trying to pinch together the plastic shelving supports when the pain pulls sharp from the back of my neck, up over my skull, and to the tip of my forehead. I pause, waiting to see if this is a brief spike or a lasting one. I set the pieces down and stretch my neck left then right, trying to loosen whatever is suddenly tight. I straighten my back, rolling my shoulders one by one.

Damn it.

I can't even do the most basic things without my body resisting.

I feel the familiar swell, like a knotted ball of anger and sadness and fear, rising in the back of my throat. I hate this. I wasn't doing anything wrong, so why is my body punishing me like this? I am angry because I am powerless to change the thing that needs changing. How am I going to take care of a baby when I can't even assemble a shelving rack? I push the rack aside and press my hands into my knees. When traced past its surface expression and to the center of its core, anger illuminates. It clarifies that which we most desperately want to protect. My vision blurs as my eyes fill with tears. Anger signals that we are incapable of control, unable to protect that which is most precious, most vital to our being. Anger is not only an emotion, it's a clue something is wrong, that the equilibrium has shifted perilously.

I move, slowly, awkwardly, so that I can lie on the ground, one arm curled under my head, the other circling my belly; the shelving unit scattered around me like a disassembled nest.

Every time I try to make progress I am stalled by pain.

My head aches. I have a headache. Ache. There is that word again.

To ache is to recognize a need.

But what is it that I need?

He

He tells me it is hard to know how to enter into pain that is so isolating. How can you be close, he wants to know, to someone who has this thing that is inherently distancing inside her body? He tells me how sad it makes him to watch me, someone he loves, be in so much physical pain and not be able to do anything about it. He tells me he feels helpless. He tells me he is afraid.

I purchase, wash, dry, fold, then put away a collection of small white onesies. We dismantle the double bed in the guest room, move the mattress to the basement, and reassemble a crib in its place. We place a bookshelf next to an old blue rocking chair and line it with books, a basket of infant toys, a basket of burp rags. We buy diapers. We buy wipes. Those who love us host baby showers after which we are sent home with blankets and bottles and picture albums.

My belly expands into a smooth orb below my breasts. The baby is in a position where it kicks, with regularity and surprising force, at the ribs on my right side. I eat grapefruit every day. I sleep with one pillow between my knees and another behind the small of my back. I attend a birthing class on Saturday mornings at a yoga studio where we practice mindfulness and breathing techniques and hypnosis. I read Ina May Gaskin and write a birth plan. *Medication only if and when I request it. Place baby on my chest immediately following the birth, skin to skin.*

As if worried the thoughts alone may be contagious, I write my fears on a separate sheet. *I am afraid labor will make the pain worse, not just during the birth but permanently. I am afraid the pain will force me to need extra medication and intervention. I am afraid I will have a stroke. I am afraid the pain will be so severe I won't be able to mother an infant.*

How much pain can you handle?

Then again, not everything born of brokenness is itself broken.

Evidence: two and a half years after the pain arrived, my faulted body births a faultless baby girl. I am nothing if not a paradox.

Having served its purpose, the water inside me lets go. I negotiate my way through the labor pains as they increase throughout the day. We have language, medication, entire buildings and wards, a script for this type of pain. Labor is a pain my body knows what to do with. It is constructive. Deliberate. It has one clear goal.

In a swift motion the midwife wraps the baby in a blanket and places the bundle across my breast. Her cheeks are round and full. Her right eyelid is swollen, unable to open fully. She is covered in a thin white vernix that slips away easily from her skin when I touch her. She is content. She does not cry.

She is magnificent.

We expect our bodies to rip open when we birth babies. Doing so follows the rules of productive pain and anticipated brokenness.

I have a daughter. I have proof. Listen to me when I speak, I am telling the truth. Like the baby on my chest, the pain inside me is alive.

Classifications

Pink. Puce and Blush. Shocking, Fluorescent, Magenta.
Light and Hot and Deep. Champagne, Lace, Pale. Spanish
or Cameo or Orchid. Mimi. Tango, Congo, New York, Queen.
Coral. Rose.

A covey of quail. An exaltation of larks. A charm of finches.
A scold of jays. A clamor of rooks. A wisdom of owls. An
ostentation of peacocks. A murmuration of starlings.

Exertional headaches. Medication overuse headaches.
Sinus headaches.

Now I'm a mother.

I know how to soothe my daughter when she cries.

I continue to try and yet nothing makes the pain inside my body go away.

Traditional Western medicine has attempted, and failed, to locate the source of and the solution to my pain. I always assumed that when it came to the body, doctors could provide answers, or at the very least, options. Where there was once optimism, I now notice a resistance rising in my chest with each new appointment I schedule. This resistance has less to do with medicine and more to do with the loss of hope I experience each time a prescribed course of treatment—treatments that are often invasive or altering in some way—fails.

So far everything I have tried in an effort to stop the pain has failed. Years have passed and I am nowhere nearer to an answer than I was when it all began.

With this realization I find myself in fewer doctors' offices and instead, with a baby on my hip, in more alternative medicine clinics. Since the 1990s, insurance companies have stopped funding multidisciplinary approaches to pain management. *The law is on the side of the normal.* This means each dollar I pay for treatment outside of the traditional medical system comes from my own pocket.

I have a lot to learn about alternative medicine. It's slower. More careful. More thorough. More money. The lexicon is different. So are the practitioners themselves, the offices they inhabit, the magazines stacked in the waiting rooms, and the techniques used to approach pain. I am prescribed vitamins and detoxes, minty topical creams and earthy essential oils. Teas. I am instructed to *let go of my pain.* I am asked to ground myself through my feet and release the pain through the crown of my head. *Watch as it floats away.* I am asked about *the strong sensations* that I feel in my body. They want to know: *What is your body trying to tell you with this pain?* They want to know: *Am I buying only organic?* They want to know: *What color is the pain?* I stand straight and hold my arms directly in front of my body while a man presses down to test the strength in each arm as he says words aloud: *dairy, corn, wheat.*

I am told to prune my life of that which does not bear fruit. Exemplary patient that I am, I obey. I have done this before and I will do it again. I whittle my life to the core, abandoning superfluous tasks, unnecessary identities, any and all triggers. As I eliminate piece by piece, my life becomes smaller in confining and terrifying ways. I care for my baby, I maintain my closest relationships, I keep the whole of my existence within arm's reach. Dismantling a life is a bit like removing stitches from a hemline then examining the empty holes where thread once punctured the fabric.

You would have done the same thing. You would have done anything to make the pain go away.

It takes a few tries, but eventually she succeeds—her pudgy hand places one wooden block on top of the next and our tower grows. When this happens, when the block stays where she places it and doesn't teeter off the edge, she rolls back and claps her hands together.

I hold out another block with one hand while I press the fingertips of the other firmly into the top of my cheekbone just below the temple, the tender spot where today it hurts the most.

I should be able to withstand this. We aren't even doing anything.

It's not fair that the pain is louder than my daughter's joy.

She stacks the third block then with a sweep of her hand immediately knocks the tower to the ground. She giggles, delighted by her ability to effect change.

He is washing dishes in the kitchen when I call him into the room. *I'm sorry, I say. Can you sit here with her? I can't. I just can't anymore.*

He knows. I don't need to explain to him that I can't sit on the floor with our daughter because the pain in my head has become unbearable. In this way we know each other well.

He assumes my place on the floor as I lean over to kiss the top of her head. She is unfazed by this parental changing of the guard, her attention keen on arranging the blocks in a pattern only she understands. A lump rises in the back of my throat as I walk out of the room.

I hate this.

As I crawl into bed, I can make out the sound of blocks crashing to the floor, followed by the trill of her laugh. He laughs alongside her then says something that I can't fully hear. I press my eyes closed and drag my fingers along my forehead, almost as if I am pinching the skin, trying to massage out the pain that has spread across my forehead. I want that to be me. I want to be the one laughing with her. I want to be the one handing her blocks to stack.

But it's not me.

I am still nursing, which means there is little I can do and even less that I can take to round off the sharpest corners of the pain. I have gone, in a matter of minutes, from being an active participant to an auditory observer of my life. I am, in this moment, closer to the pain in my body than to anything, anyone, else. Closer to the pain than I am to the person who knows me best. Even closer than I am to the baby who relies solely on my body to survive. I press my fingertips into the softness behind my ear as a thought enters my mind: *It's been this bad before and it always gets better, this hasn't killed me yet.* And then: *This will never go away.*

Treatment Records: Four Years In

MEDICATIONS

Compazine (IV). Nortriptyline. Baclofen. Midrin. Dihydroergotamine. Depakote (IV). Alprazolam. Duloxetine. Topamax. Ketoprofen. Gabapentin. Ibuprofen.

TESTS

MRI Cervical and Upper Thoracic Spine with Contrast. MRI Cervical and Upper Thoracic Spine without Contrast. CT Scan of Brain with Contrast. CT Scan of Brain without Contrast. MRA of the Circle of Willis. CBC Blood Panel. Heavy Metals Screening. Thyroid. Pregnancy. Urine.

SUPPLEMENTS

Iron. Folic Acid. Multivitamin.

ALTERNATIVE TREATMENTS

Chiropractic Adjustments. Acupuncture. Cognitive Behavioral Therapy. Chocolate. Hypnosis. Reiki. Running. Netflix. Active Release Therapy. Ophthalmological Exam. Temporomandibular Joint Treatment. CrossFit Gym Membership.

The Brothers Grimm tell the story this way: Rumpelstiltskin, the mischievous imp, grew so angry when the miller's daughter correctly guessed his name that he stamped one leg deep into the ground then pulled his other leg with such fury that he split in two.

Split in two.

Imagine. A name so powerful it rips a body apart.

A single word rises to the surface: *soon.*

Woven fibers from the carpet impress semicircles on my legs. Sweat catches in the crease behind my knees. Damp strands of hair like wet webs cling to my forehead, my neck. Panic attacks are like cruel orgasms that rip through the body, only the sensation is a vibration caught in transit somewhere between pleasure and pain.

I lick my lips, thirsty, tasting rendered salt.

How much longer? I plead, praying to God, to Mary, to the Universe, to my own body, to the void surrounding me, to the spirits below, to Sisyphus, ever nearing the summit.

What question was I asking in that moment? How much longer will pain dominate my days? How much longer until I find relief? Until a diagnosis, a death, an acceptance, a refusal, a bargain, a break?

Soon.

Soon the pain will stop? Or soon the pain will stop me? Either peril possible.

Summoned from the void, not of my own creation, as close to the divine as I have known. One word, a new name ripped from my hip as I lay destroyed on the ground.

Soon.

Claiming it was *just as faithful, just as obtrusive and shameless, just as entertaining, just as clever*, German philosopher Friedrich Nietzsche named his pain *Dog*.

I shall call mine *Soon*.

Until they tell me otherwise, until I am provided with a new script, a new language, a new timeline, relief and reprieve, it will remain *soon*. Soon it will be over, soon it will be here again. Rinse, repeat, there is no end in sight.

Pain like a shelf on the tops of my cheekbones. *Soon*. I say it again with conviction, a whisper as desperate as the prayer I want but never know how to say. I feel the space below my sternum expand like a balloon as I exhale the word out of my body and into the air beyond my parted lips. Gray cotton wraps around my brain. A scrim drops like a theater curtain. My neck is a zipper whose elements won't align. A rod punctures my skull behind my left ear.

Classifications

White. Ivory. Silver. Whitewash. Isabelline. Lily and Beige and Cream. Eggshell. Navajo. Vanilla. Whitesmoke or Snow. Honeydew and Mintcream. Pearl. Ghostwhite. Seashell. Milk. Linen. Ecru.

A kettle of hawks. A murder of crows. A bevy of swans. An ascension of larks. A siege of cranes. A wisp of snipes. A storytelling of rooks. A pitying of turtledoves.

Head-injury headaches. Menstrual headaches. Hangover headaches.

I am holding a small hooded sweatshirt, a doll, a pair of pink shoes, and the book about a feisty gorilla escapologist. Avoiding the floorboard I know creaks, I walk into my daughter's room where I hear the even cadence of her breath as she sleeps, mouth open, a soft elephant tucked securely under her chin.

I read recently that people who deal with pain have an enhanced tolerance for chaos. The author likely wasn't referring to the everyday chaos or literal mess of a home containing a toddler, but nevertheless the statement holds true.

Every day, as it should, the house undoes itself. Dress-up clothes are scattered around the basement. There are crackers and crumbs and empty cups in every room. We toss washrag after washrag into the laundry bin. Then each night after putting my daughter to bed, I wind my way through the house, returning to their proper place the pillows, the blankets, the puzzle pieces, the miniature plastic dishes from the toy kitchen. I do this, this ritualistic returning, less because I want the appearance of a clean home and more because it is one of the few actions I can control. At night, I translate chaos into something that looks a lot like clarity. A nag inside me quiets when I know where each object belongs.

All at once, inside the confines of the very same day, my house qualifies equally as two: part chaos, part order. Likewise, I qualify as two: part functioning, part pain. Ill, well. In-between. The binary is part of the whole: for the house, for our health, for me.

Friends offer the names they have given their pain.

One turns to me to say *maybe this is your cross to bear.* A silver pendant hangs just below the jugular notch of her neck.

She does not say this to hurt me. But her words do hurt me and in truth our friendship never recovers from the impact. She says this to me because from a very young age it is what she has been taught to believe. It is the hope she clings to when she suffers, when she feels lost, alone, or hurt. In a way, I admire her clean devotion. She loves Jesus Who Died On The Cross For Her Sins.

I am not interested in a God who assigns crosses to bear. Nor do I desire the company of friends who are incapable of empathy. If anything, if pressed, I would say that I am interested in a God who has the capacity to absorb pain. I mean this literally, not figuratively. I mean for this to happen now, today, not in some far-off kingdom come.

Hypothesized Internal Monologue of Said Friend

She could learn from this if she wanted to because God never gives us more than we can handle and even when we are given a handful God is there in the mess with us helping us through and showing us His grace and allowing us to draw closer to Him because any pain we experience is just a gift that God uses to bring us closer because His death was more painful than anything we could ever know because in the end which is oh so near every tear will be wiped away and there will not be there will not be no there will not be any more suffering

He

He tells me it is hard to know anymore where the pain is part of me and where it isn't. He tells me he doesn't feel like he can ask anything of me when he knows I am already dealing with so much. He says it's hard to watch the life we envisioned change because of something outside of our control. He says it's hard to know what we can do in our lives when we don't know what to do with the pain.

Exist in the margins of your life. What do you see? Tell me. Write down the questions so you will remember.

For the briefest of moments, a flash of light illuminates the backyard, calling forth the garage and the trees from the darkness. The slow roll of thunder calls in the not-too-distant sky. It's early morning. I am alone on the screened-in back porch waiting for the storm.

How did I become this fractured?

I twist my wedding ring. It is more oval than round. My body doesn't even hold circles properly. I am perpetually, hopelessly in-between.

Will I always hurt like this?

The glass on the back door is smudged with prints I won't clean away. Crumbs collect below the chairs. The paint bubbles from trapped moisture. Shoes collect in a messy pile by the back door. Reduction magnifies disorder. This is what it feels like to live a small life. There is a peculiar opportunity to be found within constraint.

Soon.

Pain slows the world. It changes what I see.

Which is louder, me or the pain?

It rearranges not just the actions of my days but the words in my mind. It dictates what is possible. What I now know to expect. It's been four years.

Should we have another baby?

It's the end of summer. That stretch of August in Iowa where the humidity is so thick it feels as though you can lift it with your hands. Another flash of lightning reveals the dahlias. They have bloomed in force this year, wide tubes of yellow rising tall next to the coneflowers. In the garden, carrot tops begin to topple. The compost threatens to overflow the bin.

A flash then a roll.

Why is it that I control nothing?

The pause of the moment is hypnotic. I will remember this. I will remember how I am cut by pain like the chimney in the center of this old house while my family sleeps peacefully inside. No one alive knows this moment but me. I hold my breath as long as I can. *Soon.*

The plants are thirsty. We needed this storm.

I live a life of uneven lines.

I take my daughter to the public library on Fridays for toddler storytime where we sing songs about farm animals. Always songs about farm animals. Every single song is about farm animals.

Like me, the parents in the room are bored, in love with their children, exhausted, and hungry for uninterrupted conversation with individuals who do not throw food. We corral our strollers in the hallway so that we can make our way—with our children our snack cups our water bottles our diaper bags and our coffees—into the storytime room. The perimeter fills first because we all vie for spots that allow us to recline against the wall.

When storytime ends, my daughter chooses board books with pictures of other babies to take home and we say goodbye to our friends. Just before we leave, we ride the elevator upstairs, my daughter proudly pressing the buttons. I don't have much time because it's lunchtime and I can tell she's tired, but still I hurry to select a few books of my own. Once home, I feed my daughter an apple. I give her sliced carrots and half a bagel. We read the library books and she, thankfully, snuggles into her bed. If it's a good nap, I'll have ninety minutes.

I make a pour-over coffee then head to the couch with my new books. I flip through the first one, stopping to read about a study where participants were encouraged to shout expletives while experiencing physical pain. *Anger,* the author suggests, *is the single, most salient emotional contributor to pain.* I read on. *Scientists have found that the stronger the curse words people use while experiencing pain the higher their tolerance for that pain.*

This is interesting. *Cursing numbs pain.* Science is working to reveal the netted relationship between language, emotion, experience, and tolerance.

The study went on to examine the social perception of pain. Researchers noted that injured patients received different types and amounts of care based on the perceived severity of the words used to express pain.

Women in pain, they noted, *are often women enraged but incapable of communicating that rage constructively.* The reason for this, the author posits, is because societal norms and expectations for women—most of which are based on antiquated notions of purity—are so deeply ingrained they continue to shape both the expression of pain by the sufferer and the perception of pain by the observer. That means that for many women, when using words to express pain, the lexicon from which they are able to choose is severely limited.

I set the books aside then walk to the kitchen. I slice an apple and return to the couch.

Am I angry? Maybe. Sure. I mean, who isn't?

I take a bite of apple.

But certainly I am not enraged.

Vocabulary Lessons

_____:

(noun) I want a word for the spot on the floor, the one just to the right of the oven, where you sit when devastated.

It sounds a bit like what happens when you press your thumb and middle finger together but it's not at all like the word *snap*. Try *aloe*. Try *breeze*. The word wants to be more than it is. It's carbon. It would sink if placed in water but I don't recommend you try it. It baffles. Press harder with your heel. Once you say it aloud, it becomes dust floating in the air around your head.

Used in a sentence:

It might all be manageable if someone sat _____ with me.

I am learning how to listen to my body. This time it knows. Even before taking the test, some deep-seated part of me recognizes the shift. I pull my daughter close so I can whisper in her ear. *Mommy has a baby in her tummy.*

When I tell him, he smiles. He exhales while pulling me into a hug. *I guess we are going to do this again.*

Unlike my first pregnancy, this one is turbulent. For weeks I tolerate only dry cereal and grapefruit, water and black coffee. I keep having to sit down unannounced—at the entrance of the grocery store, in a neighbor's backyard, halfway between the house and the garage—until the nausea subsides. The unevenness of my blood sugar triggers more headaches than usual but there is nothing I can take or do to make the pain go away. My only option is to endure it. To endure the slimy nausea that has grafted onto the already relentless pain.

I lie on my side, knees pulled close to my stomach, as my daughter arranges pots in her play kitchen. She brings me plates overflowing with pieces of wooden bread topped with slices of felt cheese. She pours imaginary water into a plastic teacup and hands it to me with a wordless smile. She asks if the baby wants fruit. When I tell her yes, she uses a plastic knife to separate a wooden apple with slices joined together by small rounds of Velcro. She brings the apple to me but, because she knows what is funny, she also puts a small felt shrimp on the plate among the slices. She can't contain her laughter—it literally bubbles out of her as she stumbles in my direction, the plate wobbling in her outstretched hands.

A seed. A peppercorn. A blueberry. A raspberry.

Naming dignifies presence. It confers awareness. It designates meaning. To name is to reflect the intimacy that exists between two parts: a known and an unknown entity.

The baby has resided in my body for only a few short weeks and already we possess an orchard of words to describe its existence to the world. Pregnancy is well understood in part because it is an activity of the female body that both men and women profit from knowing. Contrast what is known about pregnancy, a proper function of the uterus, to what is known about endometriosis, a dysfunction of the same organ. When it comes to medicine, the fervor of pursuit hinges on the beneficiary. Detached from production—or reproduction, as the case may be—pain alone exposes *the poverty of the language*. It has been year after year after year after year after year and still I have only one word, my own word, for the pain roving throughout my body: *soon*.

I want to write rage but all that comes is sadness.

Data Collection: The McGill Pain Questionnaire

The McGill Pain Questionnaire was developed in 1971 by physicians Ronald Melzack and Warren Torgerson in an attempt to
provide patients with language to more accurately describe the
experience of pain. The questionnaire aids patients who struggle
to generate the nuanced descriptions used by physicians as part
of the evaluative and diagnostic process.

Data Collection: The McGill Pain Questionnaire

What does your pain feel like? Circle the words that best describe your experience of pain.

Temporal: flickering, quivering, pulsing, throbbing, beating, pounding

Spatial: jumping, flashing, shooting

Punctate pressure: pricking, boring, drilling, stabbing, lancinating

Incisive pressure: sharp, cutting, lacerating

Constrictive pressure: pinching, pressing, gnawing, cramping, crushing

Traction pressure: tugging, pulling, wrenching

Thermal: hot, boring, scalding, searing

Brightness: tingling, itchy, smarting, stinging

Dullness: dull, sore, hurting, aching, heavy

Sensory: tender, taut, rasping, splitting

Tension: tiring, exhausting

Autonomic: sickening, suffocating

Fear: fearful, frightful, terrifying

Punishment: punishing, grueling, cruel, vicious, killing

Affective evaluative sensory: wretched, blinding

Evaluative: annoying, troublesome, miserable, intense, unbearable

Sensory: spreading, radiating, penetrating, piercing, tight, numb, drawing, squeezing, tearing, cool, cold, freezing

Affective evaluative miscellaneous: nagging, nauseating, agonizing, dreadful, torturing

The onus is on me to find the right words to properly express my pain. No one else will do this for me.

I close my eyes and draw my attention in—past my skin, below the bone, to the space where pain settles like water at a low point. I allow the words to pass through—over—the sensation until there is a flash of recognition.

I choose *Tender. Spreading. Sharp. Exhausting.*

These words have a lot to carry. They are responsible for broadcasting to the world the exact sensation of physical pain as well as the overarching experience of the body in pain. They must represent sensation as well as emotion. They are measurements of strength and perseverance. Each word has an entire life of its own, a story behind our understanding. Evidence: what is *terrifying* to me might only be *tiring* to you. It's *not only a new language that we need, more primitive, more sensual, more obscene, but a new hierarchy of the passions.*

Strung together, with their baggage and potential in tow, they tell a story that influences how my pain is—how I am—treated socially, institutionally, by my peers and my physicians. I look healthy. I smile a lot. My lab work is often pristine. I eat my vegetables and exercise regularly. I don't smoke. Because of this, it's difficult for some people to believe me when I say I am in pain. This is why my words matter. I have learned that for you to believe me I have to first earn your trust. Only then can I begin the work of effectively conveying my truth.

Tugging. Heavy. Cruel.

There are endless, beautiful ways to use words to describe what I feel. Here, listen: days when the pain is quiet are like warm peach cobbler on a summer night, cicadas singing in the trees. But days when pain overwhelms taste like cold coffee in a beautiful ceramic mug. They are a girl shuffling through the house wearing her mother's shoes. They are leaves lodged in the gutter. They are dirt caught behind your grandmother's pearl earring. Good days are like bare feet in a clear mountain stream. Compost in April. The shiver when he runs his fingertips across your skin.

But most of the time, days are a sloppy mess of both. They are in-between. Like four in the morning. Flat like the Dakotas. A rift that still echoes. The pain in my body sounds like a sigh. Like a crescendo that brings tears to your eyes. It's a low note you must strain to hear. It's a scream puncturing the dark. The moan on the third night of a fever.

I need more words because none of these do the work I need them to do. I need better words. Why do I need words at all? *Words belong to each other.* Please be patient with me. I'm very tired. Remember when I told you this isn't an easy story to tell? How it loops and stalls and can't seem to find purchase? This is when I need you to stay by my side. Don't leave just because I can't articulate the nuance of this pain. Nothing, it seems, not my brightest words, not your sincerest empathy, communicates my inner world to your outer world. Please stay with me. What people don't understand is that I am out of options. I don't know what else there is for me to do.

How much pain can you handle?

I am six months pregnant when he suffers a severe concussion. Because there is no treatment for this type of traumatic brain injury, the doctor orders complete cognitive rest. He sleeps, as he needs to, for hours upon hours in the darkness of our bedroom as his brain recovers from the impact. It takes weeks before he can return to half days at work. I mostly succeed at not being resentful. I know his injury was an accident. I understand, better than most, probably, how frightening unfamiliar pain can be. I want him, need him, to feel better, so I work to fill the gaps in our life that need filling. He rests in complete darkness. I entertain our toddler. I make dinner and wash the dishes. I buy diapers and pay bills and wrap birthday presents. His handwriting is different now. The baby in my belly grows. My body, my head, aches. He struggles to back the car out of the narrow driveway. Spring, as it does every year, arrives.

It's a strange juxtaposition to be in a body that creates one life while simultaneously dismantling another. Pregnancy swells my body out into the world. Undeniable proof of my interiority on public display for every grocery clerk and passerby to see. Pain expands as well but does so invisibly. There is no cue to alert the grocery clerk and passersby of its inflamed presence.

I keep trying to pull meaning from this pain, to give it a purpose other than destruction. I see the contradiction more clearly than anyone: even as I scowl at instructions to learn from my pain, I crave an explanation that makes it all less random. But what if pain, just as it defies category and name and measurement, also defies meaning? When I say that, it feels like I am standing on the edge of a slippery slope, as if meaning is a consolation prize I am all too willing to accept in place of source or cure. If I settle for meaning, am I doomed to a life of this exact pain? If I keep pressing, what will I uncover? My impulse is to press where it's most tender. To drill my way to the center.

Otherwise, what's the point, right?

I lie naked on my back. Needles follow invisible meridians of energy from my head to my feet, her fingers press against the pulse on my wrist. She is tall. Knowledgeable. Her eyes are slightly farther apart than you would expect them to be. She hears something in the way blood moves through my veins, an ancient voice that speaks of channels and hollow organs instructing her response. She hums, methodically tapping hair-thin wisps into my skin, gentle but firm. The table warm below, the sheet cool above; between, my anxious body begs to be corrected.

The pain feels stuck, I tell her. *Unwilling or unable to move.*

Needles in my hands, needles in my feet; around my kneecap, in my neck, in my earlobe, across my forehead, in my scalp. My soft belly rises with each breath.

Behind a closed door, motionless but for the tears falling down my cheeks and pooling in each ear, steel puncturing my skin.

I close my eyes when the labor begins.

Let's move her onto her hands and knees and see if that helps things along. Baby's heartbeat is slowing and she's fatigued. She keeps saying she doesn't want to do this anymore.

The monitors beep incessantly. Additional help is called in. It wasn't that I didn't know how to push. The problem was that my effort did nothing to affect the baby lodged in my birth canal. *The baby is not in the right position.*

Everyone said the second baby would be easier. *It's like when you take a pair of jeans out of the dryer,* the (childless) midwife said during a recent prenatal appointment while my two-year-old daughter squirmed anxiously on my knee. *Each time you put the jeans on they are looser and a little easier to put on.*

She tried the bath already. If hands and knees don't work, let's put her on her left side. He needs to hold her leg up, that's right, like that, and he needs to be firm. Hold her in place so she can push.

At my shoulder, a nurse counts out loud, telling me when to push, when to break, when to breathe. I never see her face.

That's right. That's what it means to bear down. Good. That's it. The head is out. You did the hard part. Now let's get the shoulders out. Baby needs oxygen. Ready?

Push she commands as if I had been accidentally pulling this entire time. In a rush of spent water and tears, amid the clamor of the hospital staff now filling the room, while he holds me in place, I birth our son.

When I finally open my eyes, I can see the baby is tiny and loud and blue. Someone who is not me takes him away. Someone else threads a needle and begins to sew me back together. Sutured, spent, cord blood extracted, placenta eliminated and examined, a nurse finally wheels me to the neonatal intensive care unit to see my baby.

It is difficult because of the wires and the tube in his nose and the tube in his mouth and the needle in his impossibly small arms and the monitors on his chest and the monitors on his belly, but still I take my son in my arms and am overcome by instinct. I want, no, I need to press my face against the fold of his neck. There is an animal in me that knows. I am primal. I need to smell him more than I have ever needed anything before in my entire life. I kiss his cheeks. I am entirely broken, completely whole.

I stare out the window while the baby nurses. The moment is serene. Silent. Externally, at least. *There is a childish outspokenness in illness,* Virginia Woolf said, wherein *things are said, truths blurted out, which the cautious respectability of health conceals.*

Illness, she rightfully claimed, *is the great confessional.*

The silence of the moment calls me inward.

It's raining but the mist is so gentle that it's like the idea of rain more than actual rain itself. The baby's fingers eagerly clutch the edge of my shirt as we find our rhythm of draw and release. His legs tuck perfectly into the fold between the side of my stomach and the armrest. I use my right foot to rock the old blue chair back and forth in a steady, measured motion.

He is perfection.

In the mornings, sometimes even before I open my eyes, I notice how I am already paying attention to the pain—surveying my body for its presence. *All day, all night the body intervenes.* It can be strange to wake in the same bed while wearing the same clothes and residing in the same body but feel entirely different—some days worse, others better. What happens to the pain when I sleep? Do I shake it loose? Does it go away? If so, where does it go? Does it linger in my aura? Is it in my sheets? It's early but already I can feel the edges of pain draw nearer to the center. Attempting to predict pain is like trying to focus on an object I see only through this wet window: presence alone overshadows detail.

I am empty but he is not yet full. As he releases his latch, a thin line of milk slips down his flushed red cheek. I lift him onto my shoulder and instinctively kiss the edge of his ear as I pat his back. After he burps we reposition.

These days have been trying. Caring for my body is no longer the highest priority. My own needs are quite literally overwhelmed by the very real and present needs of my small children. I feel worn. Frayed. *The body smashes itself to smithereens.* Weak and unable to hold what

I've been given on account of these insufficient seams. My body feels as though it is coming undone in an unfamiliar, frightening way.

To look these things squarely in the face would need the courage of a lion tamer.

The baby begins again.

A reason rooted in the bowels of the earth.

The tomatoes are green orbs on the cusp of ripening. I neglected to thin the wax beans a few weeks back, so now they have formed a dense curtain of green against the back fence. Does the lawn need to be mowed? I still want to put a second rain barrel behind the garage but I'll need for the ground to dry before I do that.

Even though the baby has fallen back asleep, his jaw unconsciously moves as I pull my breast back from his mouth. My temples and cheekbones are tender to the touch. The sleeping baby curls like a comma against my chest—satisfied, milk-drunk, and woozy—as the pain spreads outward and down like water, across my face, down the sides of my neck, along the tops of my shoulders, down, down, down to the very tip of the baby's sleeping head.

It's Not: An Inventory

It's not in my hair or my nose or my elbow, forearm, or wrist. My fingernails are fine. My ribs hold ground without protest. The small of my back curves appropriately. My hip bones, sit bones, femurs do not hurt; nor do my knees, my shins, my ankles, my heels, my toes.

Treatment Records: Six Years In

MEDICATIONS

Hydrocodone. Ibuprofen.

TESTS

Celiac Blood Test. CBC Blood Panel. Thyroid. Pregnancy. Urine.

SUPPLEMENTS

Iron. Folic Acid. Multivitamin.

ALTERNATIVE TREATMENTS

Chiropractic Adjustments. Acupuncture. Hypnosis. Reiki. Red Wine. Yoga. Rolf Treatments. Pain Clinic. Peppermint Oil. Physical Therapy. Spine Clinic. Ice Packs. Running. Netflix. Elimination Diet. Foam Pillows. Prenatal Yoga. Marriage Counseling.

I learn to live in the hollow.

I also learn to hide in it.

This happens when you have pain no one else can see.

Camouflaged against the scheduled backdrop of ordinary life, undetected, taciturn, present only when I lend it my voice. Sometimes this troubles me. I have wanted to burlesque the pain, wishing for a visible keloid, an obvious limp, a brace, marks where the doctor tugged the thread stitching skin to split skin. *A wound marks the threshold between interior and exterior.* I have no such threshold. I hurt the normal.

Today is my nephew's birthday. Everyone dresses as superheroes to celebrate. Pizza and also balloons, cake, boxes of juice with impossibly tiny plastic straws, odd-shaped packages wrapped in iridescent paper topped with coiled ribbon. We gather in a rented gymnasium to sing.

I take a baby in my arms and walk to the lobby enough times to raise suspicion.

You should leave. Go home. Rest.

Year after year after year after year I explain it anew: leaving will not help. There is no threshold; therefore, absence solves nothing. Little of life remains when wellness predicates participation.

Perhaps

Perhaps I could have said this: thanks for noticing.

It's not that I want to keep leaving the party, but you see it's difficult for me to be in this room. It's funny because, yes, it's the noise and the commotion and the bright lights, but there's something else that makes these types of situations difficult, too. They remind me that I never get to escape the pain. It's with me always. Whether I stay or go, the pain demands attention. But thank you for giving me an out if I needed one. I wish it wasn't this way, either. Thank you for seeing that I am hurting. I feel less alone when we can talk this way.

Is it still considered loneliness if pain never leaves?

The nurse inserts an IV in my arm. She has compassionate eyes. Her hands move deliberately across my body as she tucks the blanket under my legs with the tenderness of a caring mother. *We are giving you a cocktail,* she says. *One of these will hopefully address the problem and get you feeling better soon.*

The lights are so bright. It's almost midnight. I lie tucked beneath a thin blanket under an imposing array of lights in a curtained-off extension of the emergency room. Around me I hear the clamor of beeping machines. Someone somewhere is crying. The pain in my head, sharp like a knife, sharp like an insult, like an unwanted surprise, like terror, threatens to undo me. Why are the lights so bright?

Earlier in the afternoon, suddenly and without warning, the intensity of pain increased to an intolerable level. It frightened me that I could do nothing to stop it as it pressed outward against the frame of my body. There is a resolve to this pain that makes it feel different. Like it knows I have been ignoring it while I tend to my children. Like it will do whatever it needs to reclaim my complete attention.

I don't even like cocktails, I think to myself as the medicine enters my bloodstream and I fall, finally, at last, thankfully, away from the lights, for a while at least, asleep.

The Medicalization of Pain: A Primer

For centuries, what healers, religious leaders, witches, elders, and philosophers could not explain, medicine now decisively proves. Autopsies, testing, and surgery now have the capacity to locate error and injury in ways that lead to pain alleviation, health, and longevity. However, by assigning the responsibility for explaining and alleviating pain to the institution of medicine, we have, maybe unknowingly, reduced its explanation to a *mere transaction of the nervous system.*

The widespread dissemination of aspirin by Bayer at the beginning of the twentieth century solidified the shift in popular thinking from pain as a mystery to pain as a function. In this way, modernity has succeeded in diminishing a holistic experience into a physical one. By so successfully narrowing the definition of pain, it's possible that we have disregarded fundamental aspects of its structure. What are we supposed to do with pain that circumvents medical explanation? With pain that neither kills nor solves any foreseeable problems?

What we can't eliminate, we incorporate.

I'm worn out from chasing a diagnosis. I need a break.

If the meaning of this pain is not medical, if I can't eliminate any portion of it, then I'll have to learn how to incorporate the experience of pain into my everyday life. What other choice do I have?

I schedule fewer and fewer appointments. I use the last of my herbal supplements and don't purchase refills. It's like I need to figure out who this newest version of me—this in-between-woman-not-scholar-mother-in-pain—is. I can't separate myself from the pain; that much is clear. It's relentless and it does me no favors to pretend otherwise. But is it possible to separate the pain from me? Not literally, but as a thought exercise. What happens when I think about pain not as a malfunction of my body but instead as a certainty of life?

It's been seven years.

I tend to the pain as much if not more than I tend to myself.

Pivot.

Change the question.

Not surprisingly, the switch from elimination to incorporation takes place in the margins of the day. As I wash the dishes in the evening, standing before a sink filled with scalding water, as I walk my children around the block slowly in the morning, slowly in the afternoon, slowly after dinner but before bed—I begin to think about how pain is more than an object of disorder in my own body. It's a cryptic unknown that, in one form or another, affects everyone. It's unavoidable, try though we may. But why? Beyond the medical explanations of pain as signal and source, what is the purpose of pain? Where does it come from and why does it so stubbornly persist?

Begin with what you know.

I was something different, someone different, before the pain took control of my body. I wonder what pain was before medicine took control?

Adam and Eve: A Primer

Start at the beginning. That is, if you can find it.

The story goes that God spoke light into being.

No. That's not how it happened.

That's not the beginning.

Before this story, another already existed. There was the earth—a vast, wasted space, a desolate barrenness. There was water, dark and deep. There was wind. Creation as presented in the biblical text did not occur on an entirely blank slate because elements were already at play. Forces were primed for manipulation. Some say there were twenty-six attempts at creation before the event traditionally called the beginning.

Let's try this again.

In the beginning, there was the earth and there was water and wind and whatever debris remained from the prior twenty-six attempts. Creation, it seems, is a risky business. Into this latest beginning, God spoke light into being. Then God said there should be a vault to separate water from water. Next God said land, God said sea, God said plants and trees. The sun, also the moon. Animals. And then God's likeness became flesh: male, then, decidedly, female. Naming, this account would have us believe, is antecedent to creation.

Now let's talk about the second creation story.

The first creation story, the elemental one, whose authorship is attributed to, by best guess, a sixth-century priest, was crafted for an audience of exiled people. It was designed to inspire hope while reminding the displaced of God's goodness. Though chronologically later in the narrative, the second creation story is generally regarded as more ancient than the first. The second creation story, whose author makes the case for humility, offers a closer look at the origin of pain through the story of the first male and female.

Formed from the dust of the ground with the breath of life breathed into his nostrils: Adam. Formed from Adam's rib: Eve. Pause. Introduced here is the subtle acknowledgment that even God is not enough for humankind. From the start, the humans God created needed something they did not have. Humans were fashioned with an inherent deficit.

Idle and idyllic, the shameless two wandered a garden next to the place where God lived. (Yes. Lived.) Two trees had been planted in the center of the garden: the tree of life (read: immortality) and the tree of the knowledge of good and evil. *The day you eat from that*, God (foreshadowing) said in regard to the tree ripe with both fruit and expansive knowledge, *you are surely doomed to die*. Then there was the talking, vertically erect serpent. (Yes.) Then the abhorrent desire for knowledge. Next the taking, the eating, the feeding, the awareness, the sentence. Enter: pain.

In opposite order of their occurrence, God penalizes the errant three. First, the serpent is cursed. He is demoted from his upright status and made to crawl on his belly in the dirt. The woman is punished with increased pain in bringing forth children as well as an increase in desire for her husband. (Curious.) The man is told the physical labor required to procure food will similarly intensify. Pain, then, according to this story, is a consequential punishment for

Eve's disobedience. It's what all of humanity for all of time gets because she broke the rules.

But wait. It says her pain will increase. For something to increase it must already exist. (Twenty-six prior attempts.) Even within this story it's impossible to identify the origin of pain. The meaning, or shall we say the consequence, of pain is clear, but the source isn't.

I recognize the texture of this story. The roundedness of it imitates the myths of my childhood, where meaning was meant to be read into the story. Like building the house around the furniture rather than the other way around.

I want to talk more about Eve.

I bet no one believed her pain, either.

We are told she craved the knowledge promised by the fruit of the forbidden tree. What exact knowledge was it she craved? Was it knowledge that contained within it the potential to end her pain? God responded to Eve's disobedience by punishing the couple—and every generation to follow—with pain specific to their unique bodies: Adam was forced to endure the pain of laboring the earth and Eve was forced to endure the increased pain of laboring her body. Eve's disobedience is the impetus for pain.

See? Even when it shouldn't, it always comes back to the uterus.

I have birthed two children without the interference of pain medication. I know exactly what it means to embody Eve's specific, increased pain. Though different in scope and reach, I know the contained pain of childbirth in no way compares to the unspooled pain I live with on a daily basis.

What happens when we stand in the margins of Eve's story? Is there anything we can learn about pain by shifting our perspective? Let's look at the story from what could have been Eve's perspective.

Perhaps

Perhaps Eve knew exactly what she was doing when she pressed her weight forward, rising onto the tips of her toes, her hand reaching into the tree, the flesh of the fruit soft beneath her fingertips. What if she trembled anyway with the fear that accompanies risk? What if the consequence of Eve's action was not disobedience but freedom from a ripe pain hidden in her body? Go further. Press your way into the story. Things are rarely as they seem. There is so little that we know to be true in this life. What if we rewrite the narrative in a way that gives room for the fullness of existence? What happens when you take it all apart? What remains? Trees could be options, not tests. What if Eve needed out and this was her way? What if everything we encountered, objects and instances as ordinary as fruit on a tree, held the power to transform life as we know it?

Objects and Instances Primed for Pain

The lowest fruit, heavy and expectant, dangling on an outstretched branch. The red-hot burner on an electric stove. Flu shots. Uneven sidewalks. The way he looks at you. Stairwells with abruptly low-hanging ceilings. A single sheet of paper. Salt. The plastic stirrups at the end of the examination table. Potluck dinners. The volume button. The sharp edge of your desk. Mothers. The nick from a razor. That first drink. That next drink. Unprotected skin on a sunny summer afternoon. Fingers resting in a doorjamb. Bare light bulbs. A bowl of summer cherries: tart, possible, contained. A fleck of dirt caught in your eye. The first day of middle school. The anniversary. Red-eye flights. A splintered railing. A half-frozen pond.

Eve wasn't the only one to harness power through fruit.

Eris was the Greek spirit of strife. She was sinister and mean—characteristics that suited her companionship with Ares, the god of war. Eris had at her pleasure the golden apple of discord that she would toss into crowds—intentionally, with malice masked as carelessness—to instigate conflict. Her offense, and subsequent scorn, at not being invited to the wedding of Thetis and Peleus is the basis for the tale of Sleeping Beauty.

As gods and goddesses were wont to do, Eris had many children. Three of which came to be known as the Algea. The Algea were spirits of both physical and mental pain and suffering and are best described as the personifications of sorrow: Lype, the personification of pain, grief, and distress; Ania, the personification of distress, sorrow, and boredom; and Achus, the personification of anguish.

Haven't we heard this story before? The one where we wind our way back to the beginning only to find a woman holding an apple?

Clinical Documentation

SYSTEMS REVIEW

Constitutional: Lightheadedness

Skin: Negative

Eyes: Negative

ENT: Negative

RESP: Negative

CV: Negative

GI: Negative

Musculoskeletal: Negative

NEURO: Pain, headaches

HEME/LYMPH: Negative

PSYCH: Sleeping difficulty

GYN: Last PAP smear / pelvic exam > 1 year;
  last mammogram: Never

GU: Negative

ENDO: Negative

Communicable disease: Negative

Male: No

Other symptoms not listed: Yes

SOCIAL HISTORY

Relationship status: Married

Level of education: Postgraduate

Employment status: Unemployed

Feels afraid in own home: No

Fearful for own safety: No

HABITS

Tobacco, current use: Never

FAMILY HISTORY

Father: Father alive

Mother: Mother alive

Siblings: Two sisters alive

Grandparents: Alive and deceased

The Theology of Pain: A Primer

The tradition known as Christianity has historically interpreted pain three ways: as a result of sin, as a stimulus for virtuous behavior, and as a means of salvation.

Pain as a result of sin: this cause-and-effect argument is premised on pain as the result of both personal and corporate sin. We covet, we harm, we steal, we abandon, we worship, we curse, we mar—all of which are intrinsic behaviors inherited from our exiled kin, Adam and Eve. The broken world we inhabit—filled with pain and suffering, sin and death—is of human, not divine, making. The seed from that once ripe Edenic fruit is indelibly lodged in humanity. Any pain we have is our own fault.

Pain as a stimulus for virtuous behavior: as a patient and loving parent responsible for rectifying wayward paths, so God uses pain as a corrective reminder of virtue. Punitive pain is justified because the result draws the sufferer away from transgression and closer to God. Pain is an impetus of reform. It shifts a person away from worldly behaviors and patterns of thought toward eternal virtue. Pain is a teacher. A refiner. A gift. Pain is a bridle that directs while limiting the passions of humankind.

Pain as a means to salvation: pain has the power to purge the soul of sin in anticipation of and preparation for the hereafter. As Jesus embraced the pain of the cross so, too, are his followers encouraged to endure suffering. To do so is the ultimate imitation of Christ. Through prayer and faithfulness, sufferers can experience intimacy with God that both equips them to comfort others while conforming the sufferer into God's image. Believers are encouraged to take up their own crosses to move into a new life—a life free of pain, sin, and death.

To move into a new life.

I run in the mornings before the sun meets the horizon. I find the day contours differently when I begin this way. It's easier to conjure motivation, I am more awake, and there is a satisfaction to knowing I have accomplished at least this one thing.

I run for the endorphins—those delicious waxy chemicals that trick my body into feeling less pain. I run because it makes me feel strong. I run for the benefits all runners receive: increased circulation, a healthy heart, burned calories. I run because it's a productive use of the anger trapped inside. But mostly I run because it is one of the few activities that affords me complete control of my body. When I leave my house in the dark of morning—a headlamp strapped across my forehead, laces double knotted, my feet striking the pavement—I shape my experience of pain: I say how far, I say how fast, I choose if and when and if not. Most days some unknown force in my body is at the helm directing my movements and ability. But when I run, when I push myself mile after mile, sweat dripping from my forehead, off my elbows, down the length of my shins, the pain I experience inside my body contorts to my command and not the other way around. Nowhere else does this happen. In this only and very limited way, I possess a godlike command: I control this one thing.

At its root, theology is the study of brokenness.

I find it curious that I was drawn to the study of suffering before my body was in steadfast pain. Why was this the case? What deficit—created in me or inherited or stumbled upon—so urgently required satisfaction?

I am drawn to theology because, like mythology, it strives to name the unnamable. It organizes the world in light and dark, hope, forgiveness, grace. This categorization of meaning makes sense to me. Though not religious, I am deeply attracted to liturgy. I love the idea of a diverse collection of individuals rising together to claim a story that extends beyond the boundaries of their own lives. I crave the words, the images, even the metaphors, but not the deity they claim to represent. I wish I craved the deity. Remember that I tried for a while. Earnestly and with a great expectation hoping that I would find in God the focused resolution I so desperately craved. But I didn't. For me, religion was like wearing shoes that were too small. How do I explain that I have always been drawn more to the idea of it, the story of it, than to *it* itself?

The specific pain of humanity, the encompassing pain of the God who presides over all. The pain of the individual, the pain of the collective. Through text, study, conversation, and some would say prayer, theology is a quest to understand, and ultimately participate in the mending of, the brokenness of humanity. In theological terms, the precise moment of healing between God and humanity is known as atonement ("at-one-ment"). Some call this salvation, others say reconciliation. It's the act of restoring that which has been estranged. Regardless of how it is phrased or interpreted, atonement is the pursuit of wholeness.

Atonement theories fascinate me. Taken as a whole, we can see how throughout history each generation has crafted a particular atonement theory—predicated on the death of Christ—expressly designed to solve the cultural and ideological problems of suffering and pain. In the same way cultural understanding of pain shifts over time, so too does the language of salvation.

Atonement theories are constructed on two foundational beliefs: first, that the human–divine relationship has been fractured, and second, that this fissure can be repaired by a single event—Christ's death on the cross. This act of salvation is the restorative cornerstone of the human–divine relationship, yet the implications of this event and the problem of division it sets out to solve have evolved over time. Each generation has manufactured atonement theories that link the practical and existential issues of the time back to the crucifixion of Christ. In this way, atonement theories are, for those willing to believe, diagnosis, treatment, and cure all wrapped up into one.

He and I are standing in the bathroom facing the mirror.

I have taken my right arm out of the sleeve of my shirt and have pushed as much of the fabric as I can over my shoulder. It bunches awkwardly in an uncomfortable pile at the base of my neck. I stand straight, my shoulders pulled back into near perfect posture. I am mostly covered but I feel exposed. Intimacy is so vulnerable. I pull the strap of my bra down until it hangs loosely near my triceps. I reach my left hand over the fabric so that I can lay my fingers on the exact spot where the pain is worst. He peels the paper backing off the kinesiology tape and presses the tail of the tape against my skin. I remove my fingers. He rubs the endpiece back and forth to create friction so that it will stick before he stretches the tape across the muscle, adhering it in a mirror motion on the other side. Our eyes meet briefly in the mirror as I work my way back into my clothes. *Thank you*, I say. *You're welcome*, he whispers back.

These days we traffic atonement financially.

Bills from the hospital arrive in reusable envelopes. I am instructed to tear specific points along the perforated edges so that when the time comes to return the invoice—along with a check for the stated amount—the envelope can be reused. I have become fairly good at this accidental origami, though occasionally I tear an edge irreparably and am forced to abandon the recycling mission entirely.

From the doctor's office, I take home yellow carbon-copy receipts—my co-pay, insurance information, and half-hearted signature scribbled along the bottom line.

At clinics, I pay with a credit card and am given a tiny white sheet torn from the tail of the machine. I hastily stuff the receipt in the back fold of my wallet where it is mixed with membership IDs and a random collection of punch cards. I always plan to take the receipt out and file it properly when I get home, but I never remember to do so. Instead, the slip becomes crumpled, the ink fades, and when I do remember to take it out, the receipt is illegible. A paper trail of modern attempts at reconciliation.

How much money have I spent in pursuit of erasing this pain? And I have health insurance. It's difficult to even imagine the gutting—of finances, of worth—for those without reliable insurance and income. What would I give, what would I do, to eradicate the pain if money was not an option? Would I barter my house? My car, my possessions, my time, my attention? My name? Would I offer my body for experimentation, for companionship, for someone else's pleasure? Would I sacrifice time with my children?

Prescription

I am standing in the middle of an aisle at Walgreens next to the pharmacist. He is a clean-cut middle-aged man with a slight smile and sharp blue eyes. His white coat hangs below his wrists ever so slightly. We stand nearly shoulder to shoulder reading the ingredient lists on over-the-counter topical creams. Because I am still nursing, I am limited in the types of medications I can take to ease the pain. *This one might . . .* he reaches forward, lifting a narrow box from the shelf while his sentence dangles unfinished in the air. I watch as he scans the back of the box. A narrow crease deepens between his brows as he reads. He places the box back on the shelf. *Does this have . . .* he lifts another box. *Yes. It does,* he says. *Have you tried ice packs? I can show you where we stock those.*

A Theological Inquiry on the Subject of Pain

Question:

Do I believe God inflicted me with this pain?

Response:

No, that is silly. What God has the time or the desire to go around inflicting pain? The notion of a dictatorial deity with the capacity to smite each individual throughout eternity with pain is pedantic. Does God use a wand or a trident? Or does the end of his finger shoot lasers of pain onto unsuspecting creatures? Please.

Question:

Is pain a result of sin, either individual or corporate?

Response:

It's possible. Certain actions, like a row of expectant dominos, warrant consequence. I can admit this. But I struggle with the concept that the whole of creation is nothing more than a pawn in a rigged game. Besides, the innocent suffer at far too high a rate for any clear correlation to be drawn between individual sin and pain.

Question:

Do I believe we live in a broken world?

Response:

Yes.

Question:

Did humans break the world?

Response:

Undoubtedly. Look around. We can't help ourselves. Even if we aren't responsible for the original crack, we are responsible for perpetuating the flaw.

Question:

Does God use pain to correct behavior as a means to draw humanity near?

Response:

While it is true that pain may bring about change, corrective or otherwise, I can't imagine such change is orchestrated by a divine being. My life, my worldview, my body, my dreams have all changed because of pain. But are these changes corrective? Do they entice me toward a divine being? I have no interest in drawing near to a god who would coerce attention this way, who would use pain to lure me close. Again, I have no desire to be anywhere close to a god who tasks us with crosses to carry. Surely a god with this degree of power has other toys to play with. Why not pull me close with wonder? With incalculable joy? Desire. Is pain truly the only way to garner attention? This restriction of choice ought to raise our suspicions.

Question:

Can that which feels destructive to us, pain, for instance, be an avenue to better understand God?

Response:

Sure, yes. I have the capacity to take a wide-angle view on the ever-evolving story of humanity. But it's important to recognize the difference between walking on a path that is already there and blazing a trail through the woods. What I am trying to say is that there are many ways toward an understanding of a divine being. I have a hard time believing God can't use a path that is already in place.

Question:

Does God care what I think about this?

Response:

I am not afraid to admit that it might not matter at all what I think. There are surely forces and truths, realities and dimensions of which I know nothing. Claiming authority on such matters is a perilous stance I do not wish to take. But, I want to be clear: understanding something to be true and believing it to be true are not the same thing.

Vocabulary Lessons

_____:

(noun) I want a word for the longing you feel when you are lying on the couch, nearly paralyzed by a spike of pain through your temples, and you hear your children laughing in the next room.

It's a word that stretches out to cover as much distance as it can. There is a tremor in your voice when you speak it aloud. It reflects but note how it also distorts. There is an urgency to it, as though you are trying to get to the end of the word as quickly as you can. The word feels like hunger. It's as thin as a single blade of grass. Angle your tongue now and try again. Watch how it bridges in the middle.

Used in a sentence:
She'll do anything, driven instinctually by _____, for her children.

The tips of his pudgy fingers knock against each other. That means more.

More yogurt, more cereal, more banana. More kisses in the fold of his neck just below his jawline. On his round belly. On the expanse of soft skin on his cheeks. One chubby fist pounded against his flat palm? That means help. Help this shoe get on my foot. Help me up onto this chair. Help me put this round ring on the wooden pole. He points to his lips when he is thirsty. Water, juice.

My son and I share a language of the body. A signed language. A liberty taken with language. An attempt to build a common understanding between two people. Words belong to each other just as we belong to each other.

We don't always get it right and sometimes he throws his tiny body to the ground when I am not quick enough or when I don't understand what he is trying to say. But we try and most of the time we succeed; his expression of need is answered. He, we, have learned how to transmit a created language between the gap of his body and mine.

The Unknowable: An Impossibly Incomplete Micro-Inventory

Tomorrow. The motivations of other people. What happens when we breathe our last breath. Why evil sometimes wins. What matters. Our first moment of consciousness. Our last. The fluid boundary of trust. Why we even exist. If the risk is worth it. If the bottom will hold. If he loves me. If she understands how much I love her. Where we go when we dream. If the effort pays off. The depth of delight. The decisions we will end up regretting. Our ancestors. How much we can destroy the earth. How much joy our tender hearts can hold.

Can I live with the unknown of this pain as I live with the unknown of God?

I hate this pillow.

The top half is decent enough, which is to say that it is soft. An agreeable if extremely low standard for a pillow. The bottom half is a bladder of sorts designed to be filled with water. Even though it comes with a specialized funnel, I manage to spill the water down the side every time I fill it. It's a water pillow. I bought this. I spent money on it because they were selling them in the office when I was there for an appointment a few months back and the clinician suggested it would be helpful for me to try. I despise being a target audience for anything. I feel like a mark. A tired, angry target willing, it seems, to try anything for relief. Even willing to sleep on water. Everyone else in the entire house, the entire world, probably, is asleep. As I roll onto my side, water sloshes below my cheek. I have had to dismantle my entire life because of this unwanted eruption. Now I am forced to dismantle my bedroom. Dignity is a fragile flame and mine is threatening to go out.

I am disquieted. I think about pain as often as I feel it.

After all these years amid the most ordinary routines of life as a mother and a wife and a daughter and a friend living in a progressive, middle-class college town in middle America in the middle of my life, I wash the dishes and bathe the children and plan parties and paint the front door bright yellow as pain ricochets in my body between bone and muscle. Even though I often tire of it and try to set it aside, I am consumed with trying to understand, both as a personal incident and as an existential experience, the purpose of pain.

Medically, pain is a signal that draws attention to a specific problem. Theologically, it is a symbol of the brokenness of humanity. Cyclical and expanding, these thoughts tease me toward some version of understanding but in the end offer no real command over the problem of pain.

I lie in bed as the day draws to a close. Today was manageable. The pillow sags in a clumsy heap between the headboard and the mattress as I leaf through another borrowed book. Maybe it's time to leave theology behind in the same way that I have sloughed off medicine. It offers no answers to the questions I am asking about pain. What happens when I explore pain as a consequence of life? Who was I before I was a theologian? I was a girl reading myths. They helped me once before. Maybe it's time I returned to the Greeks.

Pivot. Go back to the beginning. Change the question: incorporate what can't be eliminated. Try to make sense of this intrusive force. Uncover the truth that will allow you to manage, to reduce, maybe to even, possibly, if you say it right, release the pain.

Aristotle on Pain: A Primer

In the fourth century BC, the philosopher Aristotle spoke of pleasure and pain not as sensations of the body but as emotions or passions of the soul. Pain was not included in his enumeration of the five physical senses of sight, hearing, smell, taste, and touch. He believed the heart, not the brain, was responsible for generating the sensation identified as pain. He was also of the belief that a person's moral quality could be determined by the pattern of their responses to pleasure and pain.

Stoicism: A Primer

Adherents of Stoicism, a system of belief based on logic and virtue, maintained that emotional repression and resiliency were the true keys to happiness. Through sheer will and acceptance of every situation that arose, humans possessed the capacity to overcome destructive emotions such as the desire for pleasure and the fear of pain. Stoics believed the virtuous behaviors deemed worthy of cultivation were wisdom, justice, courage, and moderation.

Those who achieved Stoic virtue were promised a balanced state of existence whereupon they could be *sick and yet happy, in peril and yet happy, dying and yet happy, in exile and happy, in disgrace and happy.*

Stoicism was founded by Zeno of Citium in the third century BC. It derives its name from the gathering place where Zeno and his followers met, a decorated colonnade sometimes known as the porch.

Classifications

Green. Verdigris. Absinthe. Kelly and Scheele's and Lincoln.
Jasper. Lime or Avocado; Moss. Gaudy. Racing, Peridot,
Malachite, Eau de Nil. Celadon. Terre Verte.

A brace of ducks. A dole of doves. A wing of plovers. A sedge
of bitterns. A brood of turkeys. A nide of pheasants. A walk
of snipes. A herd of curlews.

Ice-cream headaches. Post-traumatic headaches. Hypnic
headaches.

Sometimes I wonder: Is the pain even real? Because there are times when the pain quiets itself and life feels almost (say it!) normal. On those days, I experience an amnesia that challenges memory. It's similar to childbirth: You remember it was long and painful, but was it really that bad? You can recall the shape of the pain, but you can't conjure the actual sensation.

How can anything be real without proof? Absent evidence what remains?

There are things I can prove. I can prove the wear on my body. Do you notice how my shoulders slump forward, weighted, rounded, defeated? I didn't always stand this way. Look at pictures, you'll see what I mean. I used to hold my chin up and pull my shoulders back with a confidence that would make you blush. The dark circles under my eyes remain no matter my diet or the amount of rest I get. If you watch closely, you'll notice how I squint when the light is too bright. Sometimes I wince when the sounds are too loud. I'm constantly shushing my children. I don't mean to, but it just happens. In the car, in the kitchen, as we pile into bed for stories. I can prove a stack of calendars crowded with appointments. I can prove a cabinet overflowing with topical creams and oils. I can prove a tremendous record of prescriptions. I can prove a shelf heavy with books. I can prove files of medical bills and emails to friends and journals filled with worry.

Let's not forget, it was the Greeks who warned us of Sirens.

Prescription

It starts as a flower but ends as a compressed white pill adorned with pink flecks traveling, courtesy of a rapid gulp of tepid water, down my esophagus, prepared to diffuse into my bloodstream in order to block the transmission of specific signals to my brain.

The doctor said opioids will inconvenience my experience of pain.

The milky resin of the unripe white poppy: detached, mutilated, engineered into a small, smooth oval. A seed that knows only to bloom.

Things are rarely as they seem.

I hear a Siren calling my name.

Can you hear her, too? Cup your hand around your ear and listen. Her voice is soft like velvet. I wonder if she knew me before I was born. Do you think she would mind if I rested inside her voice for just a little bit? I can't imagine anyone would notice if I disappeared for a while.

I fasten the lid on the bottle then return it to its place on the top shelf of the bathroom cabinet.

If all that is required of me is to endure this exact moment of exquisite sensation, I'll be fine. I can sustain that much. I'm an alchemist, remember? I know what it takes to harness the power of my otherness to transform my very essence. It's when I have to live in the outside world—off the couch, out of the bed, alongside people; it's when I am required to speak and generate useful ideas, make commitments and follow through on my responsibilities; when I am expected to be a contributing member of society, of my family, of my marriage—that's when the scale tips from possible to unbearable. Sinking into the glossy warmth of pain is the easy part. Clawing your way back out is where it gets tricky.

I swallow the rest of the water then stare into my own reflection in the bathroom mirror. The Siren may know my name but she doesn't know the names of the children waiting for me in the next room. Their voices are sweeter than hers.

Spellbinding pain is not eradicated but merely dulled along with everything else and it's all beginning to run together a bit now that the edges aren't as sharp and is it just me or are we all feeling a little sleepy? This withered flower has fallen short of her potential. It's beginning to feel hot in here.

Yes, I'm sure I still want to go tonight. Give me one minute more, I am almost ready.

The Joy Plant: A Primer

They planted it near rivers.

Mesopotamians grew poppies on the banks of the Tigris and Euphrates. The Assyrians were responsible for inventing the method used to slice and drain the flower's pod of the sticky opium. The ancient Egyptians were the first to cultivate the plant to produce the drug known as opium. Its popularity spread through India into Greece, into the Arab empire, Italy, and eventually China.

The so-called joy plant was administered as an antidote to a host of life's problems. It was known to induce sleep and ease physical pain as well as emotional suffering. With such desired and pleasing results, it was easy to dismiss its highly addictive properties. Named for Morpheus, the Greek god of sleep, morphine, the sleep-inducing element in opium, was later discovered to be more potent than opium.

Morphine was used to treat soldiers in the battlefield throughout the course of the hundreds of wars that occurred in the nineteenth century. The flower eventually made its way to America, where it was planted in the fields of Virginia, Georgia, and South Carolina. Known for its ability to pacify, morphine was an active ingredient in Mrs. Winslow's Soothing Syrup, an aggressively marketed medicine that promised to calm fussy children.

Just before the turn of the twentieth century, while attempting to create a nonaddictive form of morphine, Bayer Laboratories synthesized a new painkiller (kills the pain) they called heroin. Heroin is German for heroic, which was the word the Bayer employees used to describe how it felt to have the drug in their system.

Occasionally the medicine works. It does its job properly. It quiets the nag, interrupting the pain signals so that I am afforded the luxury, for a few hours at least, of being only somewhat reminded of my brokenness.

The problem with having medication that works is that I know about addiction. I've seen lives commanded by substances disintegrate. There's nothing special about me. I am just as prone as anyone. Aside from my own will, I possess nothing that would protect me from the slide into addiction.

This is why I find myself forgoing my prescription and instead sitting in the tub filled with eucalyptus Epsom and a scoop of CBD bath salts. This is why I drape a wet washcloth over my face, inhaling deep. It's still morning. Already the pain has knotted and frayed beyond what feels manageable. Already I am less. Already I have been forced to abandon my plans for the day.

It is difficult to be steeped in pain while also remembering how well medication works. But the medication I took yesterday, the one that effectively shaved off the sharpest edges of pain, isn't designed for long-term use. My pain is long-term. My pain has no end. If I let it, the medication could have no end, either. If I let it, it could quiet the pain forever.

So which is it? Unraveling by pain? Or unraveling by opioids?

I dip the washcloth then press the steaming bundle into the center of my chest. Streaks of water trace down my sides before gathering back in the bath.

There comes a point where the easiest thing to do is give in to the pain. I have a choice. I can continue to invest the energy needed to combat the pain, or I can refuse the chase. I can allow it to consume me.

I breathe in the humid air.

I try not to cry.

One way is slow. One way is fast.

I pull back the knob until the sting of hot water hits my leg.
I try not to cry.
I listen as my children play in the next room.

Without meaning, the brokenness of life is senseless and random.

I am trying to outsmart pain. I keep thinking that if I amass enough information, if I read the right books, if I swallow enough pills and the correct supplements, if I coax my body into the deepest realm of relaxation, the pain will dissolve.

The problem is that I am trying to outthink a somatic experience.

My attempts to theologize and philosophize the pain are undercut by the experience of living the pain. Feeling it. Theorizing can only take me so far. This far, apparently. At some point, inevitably, it seems, the body reclaims control over the mind. It makes me think that the meaning of pain is somehow tethered not to the explanation but to the experience.

I remember exactly two things about the appointment.

First, during the intake process, where I recounted my medical history, he addressed my male partner more frequently than he addressed me.

Second, approximately five minutes after the acupuncture needles had been placed in my back and neck, he came back into the room where I was lying face down on the table covered only by a thin white sheet and without telling me what he was going to do without asking my permission without asking my comfort level without asking what I was feeling took both of his hands and indiscriminately pressed with equal pressure all of the needles deeper into my neck.

Hypothesized Internal Monologue
of Said Acupuncturist

Maybe she'll feel this

Once upon a time there was a girl who swallowed a pill and lay down to rest. I am the girl. This is my story now, my myth. I will write a twisted meaning into my pain.

The girl worried the pill broken. She worried sleep elusive. She worried becoming more prescription than woman.

But her worry was in vain. The girl always worries when she shouldn't and rarely when she should. She has yet to learn, even after all this time, no matter how many times I tell her, silly girl, that things are rarely as they seem.

The sensation began on the peak of her middle finger, in the softness below her nail, and traveled up her arm, forcefully tracing each vein, those branching roots of endless wonder. She felt the irregular residue of graphite as if a pencil pressed, more firmly now, into her skin, a cavity blemishing the fluent surface. It traversed the continent of her crooked body, leaving behind a mess of lines in which only a cartographer could find both beauty and meaning. She pulled the blanket over her head like a caul. The stillness before sleep is a unique haunting, for on the pitch of sleep she knew all was tethered to this tattered flesh: the body alone a connective tissue binding the broken to the complete.

Interlude: When the Heart Breaks

It can and it will. And when it does, it will whittle you raw. This is an incisive pain, both event and sensation. Wounded bodies, it is sad to say, are especially susceptible to broken hearts. The trajectory of life blindly forces you forward to the grocery, to the bank, take the children to school now pick them up. You do and you will and those you pass are ignorant of the osmium—blue, of course—below your breast. Broken hearts are quiet and helpless, tragic like dead birds on an empty sidewalk. Broken bodies are not resilient. Nor are the birds, for shame. You dream wicked as the osmium grafts to your heart—fever pitched, lips chapped, gut twisted. Of consolation is that you are no longer fragile. Weak but animated, you inhabit a life that resembles your life—tie your shoes, make the bed. You will orient to a new center of gravity, one accommodating for the density of your new osmium heart. When this happens, you may hear a ringing in your ears. It will taste of pennies in your mouth. But don't worry, little bird, you won't feel a thing.

There is only so much pain I can endure.

We take turns sleeping on the spare bed in the basement.

The Epicurean Paradox: A Primer

Epicurus stated plainly: what is good is pleasurable and what is bad is painful.

Epicurus stated paradoxically: Is God willing to prevent evil, but not able? Then he is impotent. Is God able, but not willing? Then he is malevolent. Is God both able and willing? Whence then is evil?

Epicurus, a Greek philosopher, never married and had no known children, was likely a vegetarian. He suffered prolonged pain stemming from kidney stones and died in 270 BC at the age of 72.

A Philosophical Inquiry of the Epicurean Paradox

Question:

Is God willing to prevent evil, but not able?

Response:

Then he is impotent. What would render God incapable? A force that divides the divine from the mortal? A moral code? Would it disrupt the fabric or the agreement of the world? How is this God, one who wants to make things better but can't, any better than the rest of us? Than me? Why would I rotate my life to serve a God like me? I am nothing but faults.

Question:

Is God able, but not willing?

Response:

Then he is malevolent. This one makes the decision for you. Why would you follow a God who can help but chooses not to?

Question:

Is God both able and willing?

Response:

This argument is predicated on the belief that God makes choices and has abilities. It is a human argument imposed on a divine being. It is a shaking of the fist at the heavens, trying to understand why we hurt and where the God is who promises to take away pain. God must be more than *man writ large*. If there is a God, then this is a statement I believe to be a true. That means we need to have space to accept an entirely different paradigm to exist.

Question:

Whence then is evil?

Response:

So what then? How do we account for the existence of God in a world of pain? Pain is real. Is God?

The Cartesian Model of Pain: A Primer

Descartes paints for us a picture: a boy, young in face, mature in muscle, has inched his foot to the fire's edge. He smiles coyly as if in on the joke.

A line has been drawn from his nearly burning toe to his knee, to his spine, to his brain, a conduit that distributes information through the machine that is the boy's body. The philosopher explains how the degree of stimuli (warm, hot, too hot) directly impacts the degree of experienced sensory pain (this is nice, this is too much, this will burn me).

Unlike Aristotle, the seventeenth-century French philosopher René Descartes posited that the perception of pain originated from the brain, not the heart. The body itself, and not the spiteful gods, the roaming spirits, the unpredictable emotions of the soul, was ultimately responsible for sensation known as pain.

A doctor from the spine clinic orders an X-ray of my cervical spine.

Before I leave the exam room, the physician, a short man with the start of a receding hairline, hands me two large blue ice packs to use at home. *Place a firm pillow on the floor. A couch cushion sometimes works well,* he says. *Lie on the pillow with your head hanging over the edge. This posture will help reinforce the natural curve of the spine. It sounds a bit funny, but it's a surprisingly comfortable position.*

I have lost years and thousands of dollars and hundreds of hours inside this diagnostic odyssey and yet once again someone stands before me proffering ice packs.

Any port in a storm, my dad, Guardian of the Coast, is fond of saying.

At home, after cramming one of the ice packs into the already full freezer, I pull the seat cushion off the living room couch and position it on the floor so I can dangle my head off the edge. The doctor was right. It does feel nice. I lie like this, my world imposed, eyeing the dust and crumbs and hair collecting under the furniture, night after night until one evening I forget and, as often happens with the impossibly simple yet somehow impossibly difficult tasks of physical therapy, never remember to do it again.

Clinical Documentation

Findings and impression: AP and lateral views of the cervical spine in flexion and extension were obtained with comparison study 10/15/2007. The alignment of the cervical spine is unremarkable and stable in flexion and extension. No significant prevertebral soft tissue swelling. No definite canal stenosis. Craniovertebral junction is unremarkable. Visualized lung fields are clear.

The Natural Curve of the Spine: A Primer

The shape, like a backward C, is called a lordotic curve. The cervical spine is remarkably flexible, but the compromised muscle system of the area renders it a constant liability. Unique to the cervical spine are delicate arteries in each vertebra responsible for ushering blood away from the heart and to the brain. Designed specifically for rotation, the two uppermost vertebrae are the appropriately named atlas and the axis. The atlas borders the skull and the spine. It has two arches: a thick anterior and a thin posterior. Below the atlas sits the axis. The axis has a knob called the odontoid process that rises up through a hole in the atlas and is what makes it possible for the head to turn from one direction to the other.

Vocabulary Lessons

_____:

(noun) I want a word for the lump that reflexively rises in your throat when the customer service representative from the insurance agency puts you on hold to review the notes on your claim so that you can understand why the insurance company won't cover the $524 bill from the doctor's office.

It's a round word. It has a sharp ending like a cliff you might fall off if you are careless. You must have conviction, a certain committed force, an unflinching breath in your lungs when you say it out loud. Grease on your fingers. Scratchy like wool. It is not a pretty word but it's nothing to be ashamed of, either. Try it. See what happens when you form your lips in anticipation.

Used in a sentence:
Would they call _____ a symptom, too?

There is something I should say about holding pain for this many years: it changes you, and by change what I really mean is that it transforms.

This part of the story isn't easy to tell, but it's important that you know it.

I suppose you could say that life is change. We wake in the morning where our changing bodies participate in a changing world. We change our minds, our politics, our homes, our work, our clothes, our hair, our hearts. Fair enough.

But that is not the change I am talking about. Did you notice how I said holding pain, not having pain, not being in pain, not suffering from pain? Holding. Let's see if this helps. I want you to imagine extending your arms into the space in front of your chest. Allow a slight bend at the elbow. Raise your hands to chin height, now curl your fingers back just slightly as you press your hands together from the tip of your pinky to your wrist. That's right. Now. I am going to take this pitcher and pour water into your cupped hands. Take care that the water does not slip through your fingers. I don't want to see it tracing the veins down your forearms or pooling onto the ground below your feet. You will drown if too much water hits the floor. Instead, the water will somehow, we don't know how or why or when, absorb into your pores. It will become you.

Have you got the hang of it? Good. Now hold this position forever. Oh, and remember to keep living your life.

Most days I will pour a steady stream of reflective, cool water into your hands. You will learn to hold this well. But there will be days when I will flood your hands until your fingertips prune from moisture and your muscles tremble under the strain. You won't know how much will be poured into your waiting, begging, pathetic hands. Notice how each muscle in your body is tuned to the knell of liquid? How much manic energy is required simply to maintain composure? How you modify your body, how you adapt your life? How no one can help you despite your pleas? Despite their genuine offer? Notice the focused attention you pay on not letting the water spill. It is like perpetual labor cheated the prospect of birth.

This is the change I am speaking of. It is a focused reorientation of the self. It is the growing awareness of your form as an active vessel. It is a productive stillness that is yours alone.

You will never be the same.

Keep paying attention.

Are you angry yet? I see color rising in your cheeks.

Careful, now.

Don't spill.

You are so strong.

It's just water, stop complaining.

You need to remember that this might not end well.

Not every story contains a heroine.

Classifications

Yellow. Blonde and Lead-Tin. Indian. Mikado and Chrome and Imperial. Gamboge. Imperial and Gold. Lemon. Ocher. Mustard, Straw, Goldenrod. Citrine. Maize or Medallion.

A wake of buzzards. A chain of bobolinks. A cast of hawks. A parcel of penguins. A gaggle of geese. A crèche of penguins. A flush of ducks. A peep of chickens.

Temporomandibular joint pain headaches. Caffeine headaches. Cervicogenic headaches.

I read a book advising I befriend pain as a means of reducing the sensation of physical suffering. I am instructed to draw near to the pain to more closely observe its presence in my life. I am told to observe the pain, as if one can gaze with indifference as the torturer slowly lays bare his wicked tools. Respect the pain as you would a person or an object that does not belong to you. Watch and listen. What can the pain teach you?

Frustrated, I toss the book aside. I don't need to redirect my attention to the sensation because it's already there. Pain like this is an open wound. It collects debris and is constantly oozing puss because it can never close to fully heal. I live with the constant somatic reminder that things are not and likely never will be healed. The pain I have refuses to solve any problems of its own. It serves no purpose to my being. Physical pain is not an opportunity for meditative exercises.

I understand this pedagogical relationship to pain is beneficial to some sufferers. I sincerely recognize the reflex to find meaning in difficulty. I have an abiding respect for those who can dissociate suffering from pain and am aware of the cultural and religious connotations of such practices. But I resist the temptation to make pain beautiful. It is victim blaming when the woman is told to befriend that which breaks her.

The same way I tried to believe in God, I tried to ascribe meaning to this pain. Not anymore.

Pain comes from the darkness
And we call it wisdom. It is pain.

Love: A Specific Inventory

Even when there was pain, there was love.

A friend brings an arrangement of white lilies, purple ranunculus, delicate pink cosmos. The receptionist is kind when he tells me he's sorry that he can't get me in sooner. We find a farm where we can wander endless rows of blueberries, filling our buckets with ripe fruit still warm from the sun. My daughter wears a tiny apron I made for her as she helps tear kale from the stem. I sit on the back porch with my sisters, a colony of bats swooping overhead as we laugh.

I take the kayak out on the quiet lake to watch the sunrise.

We grow cucumbers on a trellis. We follow my great grandmother's recipe to make noodles for chicken soup. A friend sits with me on the stairs and rubs my back while I work to regain my breath. We swim in the ocean even though it makes us shiver. My mother bakes peach pie and we eat it with cold vanilla ice cream for breakfast.

Treatment Records: Eight Years In

MEDICATIONS

Hydrocodone. Cymbalta. Zoloft. Ibuprofen.

TESTS

CBC Blood Panel. Thyroid.

SUPPLEMENTS

Vitamin D. Vitamin B_2. Vitamin B_{12}. Iron. Calcium.

ALTERNATIVE TREATMENTS

Chiropractic Adjustments. Physical Therapy. Spine Clinic. Peppermint Oil. Elimination Diet. Marijuana. Ice Packs. Kinesiology Tape. Epsom Salts. Running. Yoga. Water Pillow. Caffeine. Marriage Counseling.

I am to blame.

There is no evidence to the contrary.

I chose the wrong thing. In my quest to be better, I made it worse. I waited too long. I didn't wait long enough. I should have trusted my instincts. I let him press the needles deep. I thought I could endure. The enduring was what broke me. I should have been more assertive when she said it didn't look like I was in pain. I took the wrong medications. I didn't take enough medications. I shouldn't have taken any of those medications. Why haven't I tried more medications? I'll do less. I'll do more. There is enough love to compensate for the pain. Pain wore down all the love. I need to accept. I need to fight harder. There has to be a clue somewhere. I shouldn't have worn those shoes. I shouldn't have slept in that position. I shouldn't have stood for that long. I shouldn't have eaten that. I shouldn't have had all that wine. I shouldn't have hoped this time would be different. I caused this. I made it worse. I will never escape this pain. I am nothing more than this pain.

I hear noises coming out of my mouth, but these are not sounds I know how to make. They are not words or even semblances of words. I don't choose the sounds my body makes, which is another way of saying I control nothing.

It is like a fracture opened inside me but instead of something beautiful emerging, out flew grotesque moans. Redundant rage. I sobbed in my bed. I sobbed on the bathroom floor. I used the back of my hand and a torn Kleenex to wipe the snot from my face. I cried so hard I gagged.

Raw fear is monstrous. Inside of it, I am—and I'm sorry to say, you are, too—profoundly alone. There are some who are, some who try, and others who pretend to be, but I am not elegant in the shallow of my pain. I am whittled, anxious, and isolated. Alone in the confines of my body. In this way, I am as unknowable, as elusive and private, as destructive, as fully present as the pain itself. There is no other explanation for any of this.

Everyone is in bed sleeping peacefully. Their working bodies correctly answer exhaustion with sleep. I was not built that way. Or I was but then there was a malfunction that altered everything. I possess a body that has been hijacked. Pain doesn't unique me, it teases me into believing, into hoping, that someday everything will be—I will be—normal.

How much pain can you handle?

It's not uncommon to swing, within a given day, an afternoon, or an hour even, from feeling relatively fine to being completely knocked to the ground by pain.

On account of this unpredictable and volatile state of being, I continue to find the company of books easier to consume than the company of people. Books require less—energy, posturing, avoidance—while still providing what I need—challenge, insight, access to realities beyond my reach. I gladly take the small solace they offer. With only so much to give, this approach is an efficient use of both limited time and empathy. What's interesting is that you wouldn't know any of this if we met on the street. I present beautifully. I am an excellent conversationalist. A hugger and reflexive conversational arm-toucher. I laugh, genuinely, am curious, kind, and extroverted. Unless I admit you into my most true self, you will be none the wiser about the toll pain—and its bruised aftermath—takes in my life. This omission is my choice. It's a refusal that, in the end, protects us both.

At the library, I wander the stacks deliberately choosing books premised on the body. This desire to ingest the language others use to describe the function, and dysfunction, of their bodies is a hunger snagged against the edge of my stomach. Arms laden with books, I return home, retreat to the same sagging corner of the couch, and sink into pain narratives.

It's been eight years of pain.

I am reading the words of a poet, a lay theologian, with cancer heavy in his bones. I don't know this man but I imagine if we were to read the same book we would find in the end that we had underlined identical lines. He writes sharp, complex sentences that draw me forward in my thinking. His ability to rattle light into dark spaces makes me ache.

He is speaking of grief, which is what happens when pain ricochets between two hearts. He says pain that cannot be eradicated must be entered. I flinch at these words even as they resonate in me low and deep. Both reactions, I am learning, are honest. When I hold them in my mind, it feels as though they are extending an invitation to examine something I have been trying to comprehend.

Why do I flinch? Is it because this is a mystical perspective and I resist the uncomfortable suggestion to embrace pain? Such directives have always felt more suited for psychological, not physical, pain. Or do I resist this perspective knowing that when you embrace, you join together, receive into your body, your space, the company of another. To embrace means to accept what comes at you; to stand in a posture of active risk.

But wait. I check the page to be sure. He didn't say embrace, he said enter. Those are not the same words.

When you enter a place, you choose to participate, to engage, to take part in what lies ahead. You consider. You investigate. You remain you, but now you exist inside another place.

Pain that cannot be eradicated must be entered.

I pause before putting my pen to the margin of the page.

This is not the same as acceptance. It is adaptation. It is learning to sleep with the lights on.

Aeonian throbbing of thick blood through paper veins overwhelms my senses. I crave bloodletting as a means of decreasing this untamable pulse.

If only.

Such practices are frowned upon these days.

Instead, we follow a more conventional trend when it comes to lessening the sensation of blood pounding against the thin walls of our veins.

I reach to the back of the cabinet and rattle the orange bottle in my fist even though I know it's empty. It's the weekend and the pain has reached an intolerable level. It is as if I have twice as much blood as my body can handle. I can feel it squeezing its sticky way through my veins. I am lethargic. I worry I will burst right here in the middle of the kitchen, a mess of torn flesh, hair, fragments of bone, pieces of organ splayed across the walls, the counter. In the sink. I toss the empty bottle in the recycling, reach for my keys, and drive to the closest urgent care clinic. Once inside, I offer my name and proof of insurance to the bored receptionist then walk to the couch and wait. And wait.

How much blood would I have to lose to weaken this throbbing pulse?

A young and trim medical assistant calls my name. She asks me to step on the scale. She takes my temperature, pulse, blood pressure. I explain that I have headaches. I tell her the pain has reached a level I can no longer handle. I ask her to look in my chart to see the record of past prescriptions. I tell her I haven't refilled the prescription in nearly a year because I so rarely take the strongest medication available to me. *Sit tight*, she says, *the PA will be in soon.*

How deep would the cut need to be to relieve the pressure?

It doesn't matter how long I wait. It doesn't matter what he looked like or how much time he spent with me in that cold, sterile room. It doesn't matter if he ran tests or asked questions or listened or expressed empathy. None of this matters because he doesn't believe my pain is real. He does not trust me. He won't listen to my words about my body. He tells me he doesn't feel comfortable refilling my prescription because he's not my regular provider. He says people come in looking for the type of medicine I am looking for. *We just have to be careful, you know?* He tells me I should schedule an appointment with my primary physician when the office opens Monday morning. He suggests I rest. He suggests I drink extra water. Have I tried placing a cool cloth across my forehead?

Data Collection: The Visual Analogue Scale or the Graphic Rating Scale

The visual analogue scale, or the graphic rating scale, consists of a straight line with the end points defining extreme limits defined by *no pain at all* and *pain as bad as it could be*. The patient is asked to mark her pain level on the line between the two end points. The distance between *no pain at all* and the mark identified by the patient defines the subject's pain. Adding a numerical scale to the line distinguishes the graphic rating scale from the visual analogue scale.

Data Collection: The Graphic Rating Scale

1–10 NUMERIC PAIN RATING SCALE

0 1 2 3 4 5 6 7 8 9 10

0 None   1–3 Mild   4–6 Moderate   7–10 Severe

After I stand on the electronic scale, after she rolls the cool metal ball of the electronic thermometer across my forehead, after she drapes my bicep with the electronic blood pressure cuff, after it beeps, after she sits at the desk and logs into the computer, she asks me to rate my pain. She's younger than me. Her scrubs are black, the kind she must have special ordered, not the ones provided by the hospital. Her movements are efficient, rehearsed. I am her job.

It's a difficult task to reduce the severe into the specific. What I am trying to say is that the pain scale is inadequate. Even complaints registered at 10 fail to communicate the complexity of the experience. Numbers are far too linear to express pain's range. That's because pain bleeds. I can suffer hurt. I can tolerate severity. I can mitigate the distraction. It is the persistence of pain that proves problematic. *The pain scale measures only the intensity of pain, not the duration. This may be its greatest flaw.* I struggle with the realization that pain—specifically the residual, overarching effect of pain—is likely endless. *A measure of pain, I believe, requires at least two dimensions. The suffering of hell is terrifying not because of any specific torture, but because it is eternal.*

I wonder if the effectiveness of the pain scale would increase if we widened the scope of measurement. What story of pain could we tell if we considered not just the degree of sensation but also the immensity of the entire experience? Would we be better or worse for calling it as it truly is?

How hopeful are you? 2.

How would you rate your ability to choose the life you want to live? 3.

How certain are you that others understand your experience? 1.

How angry are you? 10.

Perhaps

Perhaps we could develop scales designed to measure the distance between how we feel in the morning and how we feel any given day at one p.m. Scales that numerate the times we press our fingers against the slight, pulsing curve of our temples. Scales that tally how many sips of water it takes to swallow stubborn pills. Scales that measure the distance covered each night on the mattress as we chase sleep. Scales that measure the temporal residue of anger after a temperamental flair. That tally the renegotiation of plans. Or the variation between how we say we feel and how we actually feel.

The Dolorimeter: A Primer

In the first part of the twentieth century, pain was understood to be a marker indicating the end point of overstimulation, but in 1939 medical research revealed that pain followed its own neurological pathways and therefore was likely to have its own peripheral receptors and cerebral centers. To better understand how this insight might influence pain physiology, James Hardy, Harold Wolff, and Helen Goodell established a method for measuring the intensity of pain.

The group developed what became known as the Hardy-Wolff-Goodell dolorimeter, a device that focused light on a blackened area of skin and produced a painful stimulus at 113°F. Pain inflicted by the device was measured at intensity ratings on a twenty-one-interval scale that marked the threshold and the ceiling of pain. The group defined their measurement of a *dol* as two *perceptible steps in discrimination of stimulus intensity*.

In 1951, working to assess the effectiveness of temporary analgesia, the dolorimeter was used on patients during labor. The trial observed the reactions of nineteen patients who received painful stimuli with the dolorimeter after each contraction. Patients were then asked to compare the pain inflicted by the dolorimeter with the pain of the previous contraction. Two years later, on account of the lack of willing participants and nonreplicable situations, self-administered testing of the dolorimeter was conducted by a group of anesthetists who concluded that *the dolorimeter may have application as a tool for evaluating analgesic drugs, but felt it had little application as a measuring tool in patients.*

The dolorimeter helped introduce the concept of the systematic measurement of pain, but the method was not without its critics. Henry Beecher, a professor of anesthesia, believed that accurate research required studying real, not stimulated, pain in actual pain patients. Beecher argued that any measurement of pain must take into *account all the subjective, emotional overlays that accompanied the origins of the pain.*

I read another book written by a pain expert who acknowledges that since there is no objective measure for pain, the only way to gauge it is to listen to how a patient describes it.

Trust. Truth.

I am trying to understand pain in a way that reaches beyond my own experience. I sip my reheated coffee as I curl my legs in close, tucking the blanket around me. A new stack of library books is piled high on the coffee table. My body hurts today. The pain is burrowing into my temples with a cruel force. It feels like a lash across my forehead. I look up as I hear a pop of air released from the log in the fireplace. I like it here. I have created a home that balances beauty with function, order and play. If nothing else, I can control this space.

The pain experience has three components. Past, present, eternity? Fear, hope, apathy? Inconsistency, repression, rage? How I experience it, how you experience it, how we both think the other experiences it?

We think of them as inseparable because they always appear together. I am a paradox. I am a binary.

However, we know that we can tease them out by brain manipulations such as surgery or by the administration of certain drugs. I'll try anything: slice away, insert the needle. Here, place the medicine in my palm and hand me a glass of water.

We call these three components sensory, emotional, and cognitive. Let us consider how each of them contributes to the overall pain experience. Let's.

Pain as a Sensory Experience

When the anger comes, I want to take a knife in my hands.

Vivisection can be hard to watch.

I'll use the red pocketknife my dad gave me when I was seven. As a little girl, I would use it to whittle sticks to sharp points. Let's call this my training. The blade, no larger than my index finger, rusted from neglect, dull in a dangerous way, has a tendency to stick when I pry it open. No matter. We make do with the tools we have. Please, hold my paper gown while I ready the knife.

I will begin with the heart. I'll try to leave as much working tissue as I can, but we won't know if it will work again until the procedure is complete. Muscles atrophy, you know. I will do my best to not remove unnecessary parts as I trace the knife around the periphery of each ventricle, scratching the pain free, but I am not a surgeon and this is not my craft. I will make mistakes. This is a flaw I own.

Next I'll run the knife along the delicate grooves of the spine, skimming pain from the surface. This is a difficult maneuver, one requiring awkward bending and strained arm positions, one that will force me to cut what I cannot see. Some call this faith. I like to think of it as desperation. There is a good chance I will end up slicing essential nerves as the blade dips low between the vertebrae. This is the consequence of proof. I never said it would be easy.

Keep watching. Just because this isn't your body doesn't mean you get to look away.

With precision, pain has wrapped itself like a crude vine around my cervical spine. I'll pause for a moment in reverence of this horror. I'll arch my neck left, then right, bowing as best I can ear to shoulder so you can see how pain restricts mobility. This tangle is years in the making. I feel a fever rising, we need focus. Let's return to the monster; let's return to the miracle.

There is no easy way to say this, but my head, the locus of pain, will be damaged beyond recognition. What I mean is that when I am finished I will no longer look like myself. That's the whole reason for this experiment, remember?

We don't have much time left—I am growing weak as the blood begins to pool into a sticky nimbus at my feet.

The knife will enter the temples and I will twist my wrist, scooping in a circle until the orange bone resembles an empty well. No, I wouldn't say it hurts. It's more a slow release of built-up pressure. My lips are chapped and there is a sour taste in my mouth. The knife will release the skin from my forehead so that small lines can be drawn with the tip of the blade from the socket of one temple to the other.

This movement slices the pain into manageable pieces, making them easier to remove. The knife will crack apart the cranial bones, so I can shave the pain from each jagged edge in a manner that eliminates all possibility of regeneration. The knife will sever the tissues and nerves and vessels clotted in a heavy knot at the base of my skull, leaving a clean white cavity.

Let's rest for a moment so I can wipe the blade on the back of my hand. The pain lies in a limp pile between you and me. From here, it looks like nothing more than a harmless mess of frayed electrical wires. I should have done this years ago.

I'll take the gown back now. Thank you for holding it.

Come closer. Here, sit with me here on the floor. It's your turn.

Pain as an Emotional Experience

When the anger comes, I want you to feel what I feel. I want to sit across from you when this happens so I can watch the changes in your face as I graft my pain into your perfect body.

I will watch the confusion in your eyes as the heaviness settles into your shoulders, causing you to slump forward unnaturally. I am not proud of the satisfaction I feel knowing you finally understand.

I will watch as you reflexively lift your hand to worry the knot tangling itself at the base of your skull. I will see hope leave your chest with each exhale. How will you react as the dull ache lodged between your temples begins to throb with each downbeat of your pulse? Will you become angry, too? I will need to barnacle your every thought with the reminder that things are not and may never be right. Your liver will have extra work to do.

Then I will touch you. I will touch your body the way the doctors touch me. I will ignore your pain because I cannot see it. I will tell you to lie down and ask you if you are comfortable. I'll hand you an ice pack. I am going to take your money. I am going to tell you what is possible. Hold still while I sew these strings into your limbs.

Pain as a Cognitive Experience

When the anger comes, words like *deserve*, words like *fault*, *punishment*, *consequence*, *commit*, words like *always* crowd my mouth. *Blame.* Others think in images, pictures, colors: my thoughts have always taken the shape of words.

I roll my tongue across their outlines as if they were rare jewels mined from a rich vein. Sometimes they feel smooth like polished glass. The corners curve organically and I notice a dark coolness like morning when they press against my lips. It is tempting to swallow the smooth ones but then I remember Cronus and how the Omphalos Stone sat heavy in his belly and I think better of ingesting a violation swaddled as a truth.

Occasionally the edges are sharp like what you would find in the sparkling hollow of a geode. They nick my tongue, causing a metallic pool of blood to collect under my tongue. I find these words are heavier than you expect them to be, but it is mostly a comforting weight, like that of a steady hand on a nervous shoulder. Hours can be spent absentmindedly maneuvering words from one position to the next, turning them over and over and over and over. My cheeks flush with the effort, the crease between my brows deepens with concentration. I once lived an entire life thinking of nothing but the weight of words.

When the jeweled edges meet or when they roll against my teeth or when I bite hard, cracking my molars against their solid surface, a tinny vibration erupts from my mouth. As does a stream of blood. I swallow this bitter saliva, finding it difficult to speak with a mouthful of such urgent damage.

The pain experience has three components. A holy trinity of destruction. What we sense: a clenched muscle above each ear. What we feel: rage, sorrow, blame. What we think: this is more than I can handle.

The problem of pain is never singular.

It is impossible, useless even, to only address one aspect of this multilayered system. It has taken a long time to understand that, for me, isolating the error will not solve the problem of pain. It's a bit like rearranging logs in the fireplace while the house erupts in flames. Once upon a time, back when this all began, a switch—in my body or in my brain, we still don't know—was flipped from one direction to another. From off to on. From healthy to not. The doctor told me there was no fire, there was no smoke. I needed to find the alarm so that we could remove the faulty batteries. I needed to locate the source of all this noise. It was good and well-intentioned advice. I tried. We tried. I searched with diligence but never found it. I guess what happened is that the alarm cried and cried and cried and cried, overheated and exhausted, until eventually it started its own fire.

That, or we were working to solve a problem that didn't exist.

Perhaps the fire alarm was faulty all along and we never knew it.

Maybe we needed a different metaphor. Or different words. Or different medication or a different understanding of how pain can hatch then live inside a woman's body.

I both have a body and am a body. All of life operates through this filter. It just so happens that I have a body that hurts, but it neither starts nor stops there. Because it has cost me so much, because it has caused permanent damage, because what it has taken is now irretrievable, pain elicits an ugly rage from the marrow of my bones. I am not proud of this admission, but to claim any less is to misrepresent the tangled experience of pain.

Here is what I can say with confidence: it wasn't endurance. It wasn't a medication log or a row of stitches branching like a spider across my skin. It wasn't an accident, a trauma, a mistake, or an injury. It wasn't loss. It wasn't faith. It wasn't childbirth. It wasn't knowledge. It wasn't a scar, it wasn't a limp. It wasn't a diagnosis. It certainly wasn't a cure. Rage initiated me into *the brotherhood of those who bear the mark of pain.* Whatever story I end up telling from here on out will include this truth.

He

He tells me we need one thing to get better and it never does. He says he feels alone, too. He says I'm not the same anymore. He says there is so much brokenness between us that it feels paralyzing. He says the pain and how it affects our lives is this thing we can't shake, it is always with us no matter what we do. He says we don't outnumber it anymore.

In the car, bundled, because winter in Iowa demands a response, we drive to our weekly counseling appointment. He gestures, *What is the difference between a good day and a bad one?*

The car needs to be washed. Salt and sand film the doors, abandoning traces of grainy white particles of discarded silt on my black coat, my shoes, my pants. We should probably vacuum, too.

The body is not mute, but it is inarticulate.

Lost in translation, adhered to the dome of my diaphragm just beyond the reach of breath, is a beautiful performance of immobile, articulate words. It is difficult to hear what is not spoken and anyway we arrived at the office and the counselor is ready to see us.

Perhaps

Perhaps I could have said this: the space between is trivial. You can toss a rock from one side to the other. But to measure the distance, or to search for answers in the chasm, is like looking for shadows in the dark. Trust me—I have given almost a decade of my life to that lightless abyss. You see, there are no longer good days or bad, the kingdom of the well or the kingdom of the sick. There are simply days strung together by fitful nights spinning kinetically, lost subjects of my agency. And you know what else? Chronicity has a funny way of complicating it all. It helped when I started thinking about pain like an ocean: waves crash on the shore or they remain but a swell on the horizon—present regardless, never still. I can no more stop the pain than I can ask the ocean to hold still. Breakers refuse bargains. But thank you for asking. Thank you for seeing. I feel less alone when we can talk this way.

How much pain can you handle?

Vocabulary Lessons

_____:

(verb) I want a word for the action of reapplying makeup, specifically concealer under the eyes, after crying.

It feels a bit clammy, like it might stick to your teeth if you don't say it correctly. It sounds a bit like parrot. Saccharine but not sacred. Pejorative. Bothersome like a loose button. The beginning sounds sensual but by the end feels used. Remember your grandmother? Press your tongue against the back of your teeth. Now swallow.

Used in a sentence:
The bathroom was obnoxiously full of elbowing women _____, each vying for a sliver of the mirror.

I dream, only it is not a dream at all, is it? I sit tall in a straight-back chair, hands on my thighs, as sun pours through the window, warming my legs. It is March or December or June. She is a therapist who speaks kind words as she pulls invisible debris from my aura like specks of floating molt.

Close your eyes, keep breathing. I know you are nervous. There is a door, open it. Take three steps down. What do you see?

A dirt path. Trees form a canopy overhead, light filters through the leaves.

Where does the path take you?

To water. I have been here before. This might be where I came from.

Yes.

The path leads to the water's edge. It's completely still here. I can hear birds in the distance. The air is as warm as the water lapping against my feet. I think I want to dive in.

What happens when you do?

I swim underwater for hours without ever needing a breath.

That sounds peaceful.

It is.

Do you plan to stay under?

I'd like to stay here always. I can feel my body, but the pain is gone.

Are you still underwater?

I'm not. I wanted to stay but something in me drew me back to the surface. I was noticing how the light became more real the closer I came to the surface. I'm still here. I'm floating on my back, drifting ever so slightly to the right, even without the suggestion of a current. I can feel the straight border of water against the length of my legs. It's like the water has a pulse that beats against me. Or somehow, it beats in me. When I part my lips, water fills my mouth. I feel like I can hold the entire ocean inside my body. It's like I want the water to replace my blood and reset my bones. It sounds frightening when I say it out loud, but somehow this is like the opposite of drowning.

This is where I want to stay for always. I want this to ruin me.

Classifications

Blue. Ultramarine and Cobalt and Indigo. Prussian and Egyptian. Woad. Electric, Cerulean, Periwinkle. Powder or Ice or Morning; Cyan. Azure. Peacock. Carolina and Byzantine. Viridian, Sapphire, Steel, and Navy. Periwinkle. Midnight, Sky.

A bury of conies. A descent of turtledoves. A skein of goslings. A parliament of rooks. A deceit of lapwings. A charm of hummingbirds. A bouquet of pheasants.

Thunderclap headaches. Ice-pick headaches. Spinal headaches.

How much pain can you handle?

Maybe this is where the story begins? In a stuffy, windowless room in the center of the ever-expanding hospital, a flawless physician in a crisp white coat with gorgeous brown hair tumbling down her back tells me I have chronic daily headaches.

Chronic Daily Headaches: A Primer

New daily persistent headaches come on suddenly, usually in people without a headache history. They become constant within three days of your first headache. The incessant nature of chronic daily headaches makes them among the most disabling headaches. Aggressive initial treatment and steady, long-term management may reduce pain and lead to fewer headaches. True (primary) chronic daily headaches aren't caused by another condition. The causes of many chronic daily headaches aren't well understood. True (primary) chronic daily headaches don't have an identifiable underlying cause. If you have chronic daily headaches, you're also more likely to have depression, anxiety, sleep disturbances, and other psychological and physical problems.

Providence is a paradoxical concept.

Less a diagnosis than a description of what I already know to be true, the answer, after all this time, is useless.

How is this possible?

For years I chased a diagnosis, hoping to find within it a framework for understanding, an explanation that would eliminate or at the very least reduce the sensation sealed in my body. I believed a diagnosis would provide a name and a reason the pain existed and wouldn't go away. Because without a name, the pain, taciturn and wild, was simply me. It was my brokenness, my fault, my own name. A diagnosis would bring relief. It would provide a script to follow. A community in which to participate so that I wouldn't feel so alone. It would usher change, or, equally, hope. It would replace the unknown with certainty.

No. That's not how it happened.

Things are rarely as they seem.

What happened was this: I was given three words and capital letters whose only job was to summarize a reality I already knew to be true. I have headaches. Every day. I have chronic daily headaches. Never before have I experienced a moment that so perfectly paired helplessness with indifference.

Risk Factors for Chronic Daily Headaches

MODIFIABLE RISK FACTORS
    Medication Overuse
    Obesity
    Snoring or Sleep Disturbances
    Smoking
    Caffeine Consumption
    Psychiatric Comorbidity (Depression or Anxiety)

NON-MODIFIABLE RISK FACTORS
    Female
    Caucasian
    Unmarried
    Low Socioeconomic Status
    Previous Head or Neck Injury

I had never wanted to be right, only to be well.

What if you were to open a letter you had carried all your days?

You would hold it in your left hand, the nail of your right index finger would slide between the seal separating the top and bottom folds, exposing the throat.

The envelope is empty, creased and worn. Or it holds a letter written in love: profuse echoes of the untamed soul. An index card with one word scribbled in rushed handwriting.

It is pages and pages of a story without beginning or end.

It is a prescription torn hastily from a thick pad for a medication the doctor is sure will work this time. A riddle. Now it is your medical records. Now it is your diary. Now it is your homework critiqued with heavy-handed red ink. It is the poem about a bowl of oranges that always makes you cry. Someone's grandmother's recipe for chocolate cake, grease stains on the folded corner.

The words are foreign, the script is lengthy, exhausting, and though compelled you do not look away. This koan promises illumination.

Now it's empty once again and you are left with nothing. Just paper in your hands. This is when you begin to cry ancient tears—deeply buried remnants of every wound and scar that marred your body. You cry angry, rage-filled tears that escape through vowel-shaped moans. You cry soft sadness. You are as empty as the envelope before you. Empty like a slate. Empty like a field. Empty like possibility, like range, like a worn-out womb, like rebellion.

What did you expect?

To open the envelope is to receive a bouquet of wilted flowers.

In the water, swimming, my body knows how to rotate from left softly to right. My arm, always the right one first, reaches forward, gliding through the water, on the water, in the water, until the axis of my hips turns and pulls the arm under my body, S curve, cut, pull, and with a decisive snap of my wrist my arm arcs past the soft flesh of my hip, airborne, dive: repeat.

Water is my familiar. Moving my body this way, today, feels like the right thing to do. It's been a long winter. So much has changed in a short amount of time; it is as if I don't even know what it means to feel like myself anymore. Effort and result fail to align and I am exhausted. I find comfort in the solitude water provides, the sharp intake and the slow release of breath entering then leaving my body, the methodical movement forward within a contained space.

Every attempt I make to build a life ends in ruin.

If not twenty-six, how many attempts have I made at creating a new life?

I don't know what else to do besides return to the familiar.

Lick the wound, pull dead skin from tired habits, ache for more. You don't have to wait any longer for something that will never arrive. Dive. Dive into the deep. Let your lips part. Make space for the water to settle inside you. Scream into the water that surrounds your body. If you can't release the pain, the least you can do is release the rage.

The children are at school, he is at work, and I am home alone standing before the kitchen sink full of breakfast dishes.

Oatmeal has hardened in a stubborn jagged line around the perimeter of the bowl. Juice glasses and coffee mugs and spoons line the bottom of the sink. I turn on the faucet and wait for the water to warm.

I keep trying to untangle myself from my body, this pain. It's not easy to separate the intrinsic from the circumstantial. Did I snap at my children when they spilled applesauce on the floor because today is a pain day or because sometimes when children spill applesauce on the floor mothers snap at their children? Can both be true? Does knowing the difference between the two change anything? Does knowing the source explain anything at all? Does the source even matter?

Lather the soap, wipe the rim, scrub the base; rinse, stack; begin again.

I massaged too much topical cream onto the left side of my neck and now my skin feels uncomfortably raw, exposed to and aware of the slightest movement of air.

It's possible that I am more whole now than I was before, back when all the parts fit together flawlessly. It's like I am closer to knowing the entire spectrum of capacity, not just one end of it. I have range. I know more. I have felt more, needed more, released more, kept more, cried more, hurt more, begged more, noticed more, tried more, perfected more, lost more, grown more, risked more. Why do I equate wholeness with abundance? What if wholeness is a whittling, an exclusion?

Rinse the soap from the back of the plate. Watch the steam as it rises.

Once again, I am entirely broken, completely whole.

Treatment Records: Ten Years In

MEDICATIONS

Hydroxyzine. Hydrocodone. Zoloft. Ibuprofen.

TESTS

Blood. Thyroid.

SUPPLEMENTS

Vitamin D. Vitamin B_2. Vitamin B_{12}. Iron. Magnesium. Acetyl D-Glucosamine. N-Acetyl L-Tyrosine. Fish Oil. Coenzyme Q10. Zinc. Gaba. Femigen.

ALTERNATIVE TREATMENTS

Chiropractic Adjustments. Massage Therapy. Therapy. Whiskey. Arnicare. Peppermint Oil. Marathon Training. Epsom Salts. Caffeine. New Mattress. Ergonomic Pillows. Naps. Divorce Mediation.

« VI »

Tell me the story of your pain.

Do you know where the story begins? Would I find it in the coiled fibers of your nerves? Does it leave you wrapped in ice, sleeping on the couch? Do you feel it most when you climb stairs, when you sit on the edge of your bed as the morning sun rises, is it in your head? Is your pain always? Or is it forever? Will I find it in your heart? Is that where it started or where it ended? Did pain scar your skin, is it obvious, would I notice if we sat close? Did someone else cause your pain? Do my questions inflame? Is pain your art? Is pain petulance or pyre, the death rattle in your throat, his name, the sin of kith and kin? What of its absence: Would you notice if it went missing?

It's Not: An Inventory

It's not in my hair. My fingernails are fine.

I have scheduled an appointment with a functional medicine physician.

We sit adjacent on two small, firm chairs in the corner of her office, our knees inches from touching. She nods as I talk, typing notes on a laptop without breaking eye contact.

Her brow furrows as I describe the nuances of the pain in my body. *There are two kinds,* I say. *One works its way from the outside in, the other works its way from the inside out.* She asks me to say more about this subtle distinction. I cross my leg in the other direction and speak slowly, with intent. I want to get this right. These words matter, if not to her, then at least to me. It's taken a long time to parse the intricacies of this pain.

It hasn't always been this way. It used to be just a headache. Now it's residual. Consequential. Everywhere.

She nods almost imperceptibly.

I call it structural pain when it works from the outside in. I press my fingertips together to demonstrate the inward motion. *That's when it feels like my bones are too large for my body, or when my muscles are hot to the touch. Or when my neck gets really stiff and my mobility is restricted. Or when I sleep for too long or in an odd position or not long enough. Or when my hips and knees ache from the running I do to mitigate the pain. That's what I mean by structural pain. It transfers. I don't like it, but I also don't fear it because I know where it comes from. I can point to where it lives and trace lines between one ache and the next.*

She nods slowly, her fingers poised above the keys, waiting for me to continue.

But when the pain works its way from the inside out? When it feels like a heavy pulse in my temples or a wave of nausea? I pause. There are no motions my hands can make to visually convey this feeling. *When I do nothing different, but everything has changed? That's when I worry because I can't track it. It doesn't have an origin or a cause. It is invisible but present. It rises out of me and I can't touch it. It's distinctly other, it feels impossible that this sensation can organically rise from my own body.*

When we finish talking, I cross the room and step up onto the exam table. She puts a needle in my arm and pulls blood into color-coordinated vials. She hands me a saliva test kit to use when I get home. She asks if I have had genetic testing. She tells me I can submit a portion of the bill to insurance. She gives me a list of vitamins to purchase from the local health food store. She suggests a relaxation app I might like to download and try. Have I tried meditation? Before I walk out the door she hands me a list of upcoming vegan cooking classes offered at the clinic. Because I'm a client I can attend the classes at a reduced fee.

Then again, sometimes dysfunction isn't invisible at all. Sometimes it is laid bare for all to see.

He stays in the modest redbrick home on the back curve of the old county racetrack. I move to a new home in a neighborhood next to the elementary school with an uneven front walk and well-established trees. In my yard alone there is a messy walnut and a towering white pine, a hickory, a slanted redbud, a plum tree, and a magnolia with low sturdy branches my children like to climb.

I work to find language the children can use. I say *We are a family who has two homes now.* I say *I am one mom, there is only so much I can do.* I say *Let's practice writing our new address.*

I order a bed frame from CB2. It takes three months to arrive. In the meantime, I sleep on the floor, tucking a flashlight between the mattress and the wall because I can't reach the light switch from the ground and it feels safer that way. Electricians submit bids to remove the knob and tube and replace it with up-to-code wiring. These arrive in colorful folders labeled with columns and graphs indicating price points for service and optional upgrades.

I say *I am doing the best I can.*

I stack the dishes into a new cupboard and wonder to myself: *Where is the line between sharing my pain and burdening someone with it?*

The numbers that accompany creating a new home, a new life, are overwhelming. There are sixteen digits on my new credit card. The CVV is three numbers. Four numbers indicate the expiration date. The new bank account is nine numbers. The PIN on the new debit card is four numbers. The new safe deposit box has a key and four numbers etched on its surface. I order new checks and write *Solo Account* with black permanent marker on the box when it arrives. The garage code is five numbers. The new membership number at the grocery is six numbers.

There are fifty-two light switches in my new home. I cannot seem to learn which switch corresponds to which light and find myself constantly, and improperly, illuminating rooms. I try to memorize which switch belongs to which light. I try directional mnemonics and I try labeling and sometimes I stand before the switch trying my hardest to do this one thing right, surely, I can do just this one thing right, but I cannot keep the switches straight. No matter what I do, I just cannot keep them straight.

He and I were married for sixteen years.

How much pain can you handle?

Perhaps

Perhaps I walk into the emergency room where I sit rigid in a plastic chair while cold air whips into the waiting room each time the double glass doors retract, announcing the arrival of newcomers. Perhaps my legs shake with an adrenaline tremor I cannot control as the triage nurse, a woman with thin wrists and long, strong fingers, takes my temperature, my blood pressure, my pulse. Perhaps she asks my age and if I smoke and if I have ever been treated for pain as it presents in women's bodies?

My children settle into the oversize chairs in the waiting room. She opens her book, he twists the Rubik's Cube with both hands as though wringing out a wet cloth, his concentration instant and unshakable. *Did you know the Spanish word for waiting and hoping is the same, so why couldn't we call this the hoping room, or would that be too depressing?* We wait. We hope.

Be good, I tell them, giving them my best half-smile, half-stern look as I close the door behind me. It is a familiar routine for us all, though I do my best to schedule the biweekly appointments when they are at school. I suspect we talk about pain more than most families with young children. They know when they walk into a room that the smell of peppermint is my tell, alerting anyone near me that I am hurting. They know it's difficult for me to listen to loud music in the car. They know I see the chiropractor because she helps my body hurt less. They offer grace I don't deserve when I apologize for being short, for yelling, for not being better because the pain is overwhelming my ability to be a good mom. But more salient than any conversation we have, they see, plainly without anyone having to tell them, the toll pain takes on me. On us. I don't know how else to prepare them for the terrible things that lie ahead except by allowing them honest glimpses into the reality of my own struggles.

We wait. We hope.

My chiropractor is as kind as she is beautiful. She is confident in her height. She moves with purpose and strength. I update her on how I have felt since my last appointment. *It's been a difficult week,* I say. *The headaches have been stronger in the morning. I am sore here. Here, here, and here. Here, too.* She nods and, with the perfect balance of tenderness and strength, helps me onto the table, where I assume the necessary defenseless position: face down, back unprotected, neck bare. The vulnerability of this posture wipes away any sense of composure I pretend to have. I can't contain the sadness any longer.

She pauses. She holds my hand while I cry. *Tell me.*

I am just so tired of always being in pain.

She waits for my breathing to steady itself. This takes a long time but she doesn't rush me. She brings me tissues. When my breathing eventually calms, she adjusts my body, pressing muscles this way then that way, she rubs oil on my temples. We make a plan for me to come back next week and she gives me a hug as I open the door to leave. As I step through the doorway, my children's eyes rise to meet mine, and they recognize immediately that I have been crying. My boy slides off the chair and comes to my side, where he wordlessly hugs my leg. My girl, assuming responsibility for the situation, gathers her book, the toys her brother abandoned haphazardly around the room.

We wait. We hope.

If hope is the feeling that what is wanted can be had, then it follows that hopelessness is a feeling that what is wanted cannot be had.

I still have headaches. It requires an immense courage to continue to try, a decade later, new treatments that address this particular physical and emotional pain. Summoning the strength to try again (*That's right, take the pills twice a day for a month, but take them with food because they will upset your stomach*), again (*She is accepting new patients but there isn't an opening in the schedule for another eight months*), and again (the doctor who looks at me askance while saying, *It's funny because you look healthy but you're not*). This fortitude has nothing to do with the taxing treatment options themselves. I can withstand needles and manipulations and medication side effects with herculean strength. It's hope I struggle to maintain.

I had hope once. It was a whorl of possibility spinning below my sternum. I approached each new doctor, each medication, treatment plan, lifestyle change, each loss with hope that it would at the very least lessen, if not solve, the pain. Occasionally there was temporary relief. Mostly, there was silence. I have amassed quite the testament to my labor. But slowly, like water evaporating into thin air, hope no longer exists where it once did. I imagine if you were to turn me inside out and examine the floor of my sternum, you would see the delicate lines like a fossil where the whorl once pressed its mark into my body. You could trace your fingers along the groove. I imagine it would be a pleasant, soothing sensation for both of us.

I have seen hope alive in others. It acts as an admirable shield guarding against disappointment with a silent, restorative force. It is beautiful to behold. But for hope to continue, for its expression to be honest and true, the expectations it raises must, at some point, be fulfilled. The bottom can't always be dropping out; there must be patches of solid ground on which to rest.

What frightens me more than anything else is that I will carry this for always. If I struggle now, what will happen when I age and my body begins to naturally deteriorate? How can I possibly endure the natural course of life when I am already debilitated?

I still hope for many things—that my children will know joy to the core of their bones, that kindness will always prevail, that love will fill the rooms of my home, that someday I will finally learn how to bake a pie—but I no longer hope for freedom from pain.

Hypothesized Internal Monologue
of Said Hopeless Woman

Losing what an inconsiderate assumption it implies I had it then
was careless it's not like I set it down somewhere it's not in the
junk drawer I didn't leave it behind on the bus or accidentally
return it with the library books I didn't misplace it or discard it
or waste it away but I had it and now I don't so how do I explain
it's more like erosion because hope just eroded away speck by
speck or maybe that perched thing with feathers just decided it
was time to molt you know she never said it was a bird why do
we always assume we know what she meant maybe it's not a bird
at all maybe it's a beast an animal within yes erosion like wearing
away like gnawing away ex for *away* rodere for *gnaw* it makes you
think of rodent I'm getting closer that feels right a rodent gnawing
away at what is no longer useful

Perhaps

It's not lost on me that had I been born at any other time in history, I would have received a very different course of treatment for the ache in my head. Perhaps I would have had puncture holes drilled in my skull to release pressure as well as, conveniently, any lingering evil spirits. I may have had a clay rendering of a crocodile with a grain affixed in its mouth wrapped around my head with a strip of linen listing the names of gods who could bring relief. I may have been given a cloth wet with vinegar and opium to place across my forehead. I may have been spun in circles in an attempt to pull blood away from my head and toward my feet. I may have had a five-inch-by-one-inch gorge scraped into my scalp and left to heal by means of scar tissue. I may have been given nitroglycerin. I may have been told to cauterize my scalp down to the muscle. I may have been told to soak in a bath of honey. I may have been told to add eels to the bathwater.

Prescription

As I rise from my desk, the old wooden chair announces my movement to the empty house through an elaborate series of creaks and groans.

I walk to the couch and rest my head on the pillow, curling my knees close while pulling a blanket up to my chin. On days like this I am especially grateful to work from home. I don't take for granted the benefit of mostly being in control of my own schedule. I close my eyes to rest but I'm not tired.

I wasn't in pain when I woke this morning but now, midway through the day, the sensation has taken command of my body, my day. What began as a productive, ordinary morning is now a tangle of disappointment. I am angry that my day has been taken from me without my consent. I circle my options like a vulture, trying to decide which, if any, will assist me in the reclamation of my day.

It's too early for alcohol but too late for caffeine. Ibuprofen might mitigate the sharpest edge of the pain, but the relief will be extremely short-lived. Because I took my prescription before heading to a meeting around this same time yesterday, it feels like the start of a habit to take it again today. I have to get my children from school before too long, so edibles don't feel like the right option. I already ran. I reek of peppermint oil. I have no partner for laughter, for distraction, for sex. If I do nothing will the pain ease or expand?

Maybe tomorrow will be better. Maybe tomorrow will be better. Maybe tomorrow will be better. Probably not, but at least tomorrow will be here soon.

Vocabulary Lessons

_____:

(noun) I want a word for the doubt you feel the moment you swallow a pill.

The word feels muffled. It's brittle, a little bit anemic. It sounds like it would echo if you shouted it aloud, but it won't so don't try. Even if you did manage to say it, which you won't, it would fall to the ground and the sound it would make would disappoint you. The word is splintered. The word slams against your lips. I think it rhymes with stepmother.

Used in a sentence:

Alone in the bathroom, the glass of water still in her hand, she stares at her reflection in the mirror as _____ rises like anxiety in her chest.

Prescription

For how many years have I been ingesting pain medication that has been tested exclusively on male bodies?

Classifications

Red. Incarnadine. Crimson or Carmine or Cardinal. Ruby and Imperial. Indian, Spanish, Morocco; Rust. Fire Engine. Chili or Lust. Cornell and Madder. Blood. Cochineal, Cherry, Grenadine, Pomegranate. Coquelicot. Poppy.

A building of rooks. A chattering of chicks. A fall of woodcocks. A party of jays. A wedge of swans. A cover of coots. A rookery of penguins. A hedge of herons.

Altitude headaches. Hemicrania continua headaches. Ocular headaches.

He

He tells me that since we don't live together anymore it's easy to forget how much pain I am in now that the daily reminders are gone. He tells me he sees the loneliness of my pain in my eyes when he picks up the kids on Sunday mornings. He sees it when I say how he still knows the extent of the pain more than anyone else. He tells me he can see how I have built an extensive tool kit to help ease the pain. He says he still doesn't know how to shield the kids from the pain when he is not there to help when things feel unmanageable. He tells me he sees, as the years go on, the cost on my body and the weight of the pain I carry.

Providence is a paradoxical concept.

Prescription

What would happen if I ingested pills tested exclusively on female bodies?

_____: A Primer

In 20__, _____ _____ received record-setting funding from the Food and Drug Administration to conduct a series of clinical trials aimed at better understanding the effectiveness of pain medication exclusively developed for and tested on females. The study sample consisted of chronic pain patients from twenty-two countries between the ages of 14 and 66 who had been living with pain for __ to __ years. Participants in the randomized double-blind study were asked to _____ and then ___. From this, _____ concluded that when ____ enters the bloodstream, _____ occurs at a rate of __ per __. This insight is what allowed ____ to see that _____ impacts pain perception in females, sometimes at a __ percent rate higher than previously understood.

_____'s groundbreaking work revealed _____, which has transformed the assessment, diagnosis, treatment, and cure of chronic pain.

Love: A Specific Inventory

Even when there was pain, there was love.

A domed alcove in a historic church, red candles flickering nearby, I kneel as the octogenarian places one crooked hand on my head while the other rubs the symbol of the cross on my forehead with oil from a thimble-sized vessel. She speaks my name into a blessing of peace.

I gather around a table of food with my dearest friends. After injecting a steroid shot in my leg, the nurse turns off the lights, closes the blinds. Snow falls to our knees; friends clear it away before the sun rises. My father and I walk the bank of the river, a convocation of bald eagles lining the bare limbs of the trees. We swim in the lake after dark, fireflies dancing along the narrow beach. I am gifted an earthen kintsugi bowl that fits in my palm, a flash of gold tracing its jagged scar.

Neighbors bring bread. Neighbors bring soup and cookies and beer. Neighbors bring daffodils and baskets of popcorn and candy on May Day. Neighbors bring honey from the hive and strawberries from the garden.

Treatment Records: Twelve Years In

MEDICATIONS

Hydrocodone. Zoloft. Hydroxyzine. Cyclobenzaprine. Ibuprofen.

TESTS

Cardiometabolic Assessment. Diabetes. Autoimmune Assessment. Thyroid. Hormone Panel. CBC. Immunoglobulin A Blood Test. Lyme Disease. Rickettsia Test. Iron Panel.

SUPPLEMENTS

Iron. N-Acetyl Cysteine. Methyl B_{12}. Methyl Folate. Magnesium. Coenzyme Q10. Vitamin D. Fish Oil. Zyflamend. Ferritin. Melatonin.

ALTERNATIVE TREATMENTS

Chiropractic Adjustments. Massage Therapy. Therapy. Red Wine. Edibles. Whiskey. Functional Medicine. Peppermint Oil. Arnicare. Heating Pads. Ice Packs. Amazon Prime. Epsom Salts. Yoga. Running. CBD. Caffeine. Elimination Diet. Paroxysms.

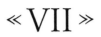

Vocabulary Lessons

_____:

(noun) I want a word for the tipping point when pain transforms from a symptom into its own disease.

It's a wisp of a word. So unassuming in its simple delicacy you might miss it if you aren't paying attention. It's estranged. Stop crying about it, the word doesn't care what you think. The word is destruction. The word sounds like humility. It feels like an orb. The word is hot to the touch. It will remind you of middle school. Try not to blink when you say it out loud.

Used in a sentence:
No one knows for sure, but _____ probably happens at night when everyone is sleeping, on a Monday, no less.

On a sunny Saturday morning, we gather snacks and water bottles, toys and books for the car ride. I pour steaming coffee into a travel mug, pack my children into the back seat, and drive to a quiet town just over an hour away to see an art exhibit.

We arrive moments after the sleepy college student unlocks the front doors. I hear the percolation of coffee in the open office nearby. We have the space entirely to ourselves. We, my children and me, this young man, are the only ones in the building.

The artist Anna Cowley Ford, whose work we have come to see, suffers from chronic migraines. The exhibit presents a series of ceramic busts that visualize the hidden pain of the symptoms associated with migraine. Though consistent in form—the busts are fashioned from a rubber mold cast taken directly from the artist's body—each bust represents, in name and detail, one particular experience, or symptom, of migraine pain. The busts are beautiful. They are also disturbingly graphic. They bear unassuming but descriptive titles such as *Nausea* and *Clenched Teeth* and *Fatigue* and *Depression*. It's not until the moment we walk into the gallery that I realize I have brought my children into what looks like a room filled with heads mounted on stakes.

As we enter the gallery, there is an art cart filled with markers and crayons and string. There are small bowls of pins. Nails. Fake plastic capsules. Metal plates. Something that looks like a chain from a bike. The busts are grouped in five small pods near the middle of the room, leaving two blank walls covered from floor to ceiling in long strips of white paper. There is a sign that invites visitors to use the white space and the materials provided to share their own experience with invisible illness. Without hesitation, driven by either discomfort or recognition, my children turn instantly to the cart, their small fingers exploring the materials as I make my way slowly, deliberately through the room.

I don't have migraines, but I know this pain.

My children are patient. They know to honor this still communion of truths.

Having woven in and out of the various pods, having stood motionless before the most familiar representations of my own pain, I circle back to the cart. My children have gathered into a small pile the materials they want to use. They carefully place the pins and crayons in my hand and we walk to a blank space on the wall. I use a blue crayon to trace the outline of my daughter's body. *I'll show you where it hurts on mommy*, I say as I gather the sewing needles in my palm. My son helps me push the needles into the space on the outline where temples would be. I pin a flat red metal plate across the forehead. Each child takes a crayon and reinforces the lines down the neck and across the base of the shoulder. They have seen how I press my fingers into my forehead, behind my ears, at the back curve of my jaw, down the sides of my neck, and across my shoulders. They are familiar with where pain lives in my body. I like to think I equip my children to encounter the unknown by allowing them to see the vulnerability with which I attend to my own brokenness. Working together, mostly in silence, using only the materials available to us, moments before we leave the gallery in search of doughnuts and coffee, we, together, make visible—we articulate—my pain onto a blank surface.

Chronic Pain: A Primer

Chronic pain is a common condition affecting more than three million Americans each year. You can diagnose yourself with the condition if you have persistent pain in the body that lasts for weeks to years. Treatments can help manage symptoms but will not cure the problem. These treatments include medications, acupuncture, electrical stimulation, cognitive behavioral therapy, and surgery. Chronic pain can interfere with your daily life, keeping you from doing the things you want and need to do. It can take a toll on your self-esteem and make you feel angry, depressed, anxious, confused, and frustrated. The link between emotions and pain can create a cycle because when you hurt, you're more likely to feel depressed. Depression can make your pain even worse. The link between depression and pain is often why doctors use antidepressants as one treatment for chronic pain. These drugs can help with both the pain and the emotional strain it causes. Pain also interferes with sleep and raises your stress levels. Both a lack of sleep and more stress can make your pain feel stronger.

When it started, I had one version of pain—the original one, the ache like a bruise that spread across the left side of my head. To that was added a second version of pain—the part that reverberated like a hollow drum, the consequence of the lumbar puncture. Remember when I told you that this is a story that doesn't end? Now there is a third version of pain—chronic pain.

In bodies that have chronic pain, the central nervous system has become hypersensitive. It generates pain messages in response to stimuli that, in other non–chronic pain bodies, typically would not produce pain. People in chronic pain don't just experience pain constantly or all the time like the name suggests (though they may). They experience pain *differently*. When it comes to interpreting pain signals, their bodies have, in a sense, been rewired. Their bodies magnify the slightest discomfort. They quicken the time it takes to respond and elongate the time it takes to recover. Bodies in chronic pain transfer sensations with what in any other situation could be called elegance. This is one of the reasons why pain medication designed to alleviate acute episodes (common tension headaches, muscle aches, minor joint pain) fails to provide any relief for bodies awash in pain.

Objects and Instances Primed for Chronic Pain

Changes in weather. Heightened stress, anxiety, and worry. Panic attacks. Insomnia. Foods with the known potential to inflame include processed meats, sugars, gluten, soybean and vegetable oil, and processed foods such as chips and crackers. Catastrophic thinking. Exhaustion, overexertion, but also the lack of proper physical activity. The common cold. Poor posture. Incorrect footwear. Hormonal changes resulting from menstruation. Repression. Isolation. Vulnerability. Hopelessness. Bright lights. Changes in medication. Fridays.

The problem with this story is that it has never been entirely clear where it will go.

Here is what I do know: I know that pain creates a fault. A rift in an otherwise seamless life. When faults like this emerge, our instinct is to fill that gap so that we are not constantly tripping into the abyss. We do this by collecting stories that imbue blank spaces with meaning. We stack answers like bricks against a crumbling facade, like bandages over split skin. We speak in metaphors. We give words to experiences that transcend language. I know that still, after all this time, I don't have satisfying answers. Instead, I have chosen to fill the space with questions. In place of certainly I possess curiosity. It's not a bait and switch. It's neither a fair nor an easy trade. It's possible I'll regret this decision.

I know that most of the time, pain is worse on the bookends of the day. I know it is not caused by injury or illness or infection. I know that it was necessary for me to explore pain as a subject of thought, a philosophical and theological riddle, not only as an existential experience. I know my body is extraordinarily adaptable. Pain touches each part of my life. It changes how I mother my children. What I can achieve. I know my understanding of pain is paradoxical. I know it is incomplete, full of craterous holes and stubborn contradictions.

Medically, the purpose of pain is to direct attention toward an underlying problem. For some people, pain is a portal to the divine, a path toward something, or someone, with the capacity to acknowledge, mend, or even transform brokenness into beauty. Theologically, pain is a useful, porous entity through which, if you look closely, you will witness the divine. Philosophically, pain, like morality and existence, is understood to be a consequence of life.

I believe the writers come closer to the truth. In a concept called negative capability, the poet John Keats characterized the ability to pursue a vision of artistic beauty even when that same pursuit leads to confusion and uncertainty. In other words, negative capability is the ability to hold in tandem multiple, often opposing, views. But, and this is key, the goal is not simply to hold these views as a measure of strength but to use them as the basis for creation. To make something beautiful out of the paradox. Something destructive. Something holy. To make art out of what arises from the negative space. The purpose is to let the tension of the two opposing views inform, rearrange, or focus what otherwise feels worthless.

I am reminded of the words I read years ago when I first began exploring pain as a subject. *Whatever pain achieves, it achieves in part through its unsharability, and it ensures this unsharability through its resistance to language.*

Pain achieves. It carries from one place to the next and in this movement it accomplishes a goal. That I struggle to articulate the experience of pain is not a shortcoming on my part. Nor is it due entirely to the inadequacy of language. It's possible that the struggle to articulate may in fact be a necessary part of the design. There is a reason pain resists both language and measurement. I don't know this reason and I probably never will. But it is an unknowing I can live with because in its uncertainty it nods toward a greater pursuit.

I know that part of the problem is that when it comes to understanding the depth of pain, we've siloed our thinking. By narrowing the definition of pain so precisely we've scrubbed it of its complexity. We've reduced it to synapses, to a symptom. We keep trying to simplify pain to comprehend its vastness. But what if that's backward? What if instead of isolating pain we compounded it? What if our approach was to layer, not to reduce? To make it wider, messier, more complex not less? To acknowledge the difficult parts where pain clings to other parts of the body, to other emotions, beliefs, and expectations?

We need to pivot. We need to change the question.

It makes sense that the answers we have generated are underwhelming, unsatisfactory, and incorrect because they are answers to the wrong questions. The questions we need to ask are not only about *what* this pain means but rather *who* this pain affects. We must establish which questions are in need of answers and who has the authority to provide answers.

Because what the neurologist said is still true: I do want answers.

But I don't want to settle for answers to questions I am not asking.

If I regret anything, it's that I was tolerant for far too long. I acquiesced to the inadequate explanations I was given. I wish I had known how to resist, how to use my voice and my experience to demand change. I was wrong to assume someone else would solve for the problem of pain in my body. It's a mistake I know to no longer make.

Conceptually I desperately want to claim negative capability as a centering truth of my life, but even I can see flaws in this instinct. I keep trying to make pain a subject, a complex and beautiful object to hold at a distance and observe. Except it is not. Not for me. Pain is not beautiful; it is not my friend. But then again neither characteristic is requisite for art. My body is neither mute nor articulate. It's somewhere in-between, caught in the margins, waiting. Poised. Less, maybe, than it once was, but not gone. It may not be entirely clear where this story begins, but I know for sure that this is not the end.

Classifications

Black. Kohl. Payne's Gray. Obsidian, Ink, and Charcoal.
Jet. Melanin or Pitch. Livid. Carbon and Roseman. Coal,
Midnight, Ebony. Davy's. Onyx and Eerie.

A spring of teals. A piteousness of doves. A lamentation
of swans. A mob of emus. A colony of vultures. A sord of
mallards. A conspiracy of ravens.

Rebound headaches. New daily persistent headaches.
Chronic daily headaches.

Perhaps

Perhaps one day I will wake on a cold January morning and nothing will spread across the left side of my head. On that day, I will not think of pain's intrusion in my life. I will attribute my feeling of ease to a restful night's sleep, to the hours I spent curled, soundlessly, effortlessly, in my bed. Perhaps on this day I will complete an arduous workout. Perhaps I will get sushi. Maybe falafel.

Pain stole my life.

No. That's not how it happened.

Pain stole one version of my life and replaced it with another.

Some days are almost normal.

I remember life without pain.

You were

free

I try sleeping recumbent in a chair.

If I could take it from you, I would.

If you could write about anything in the world, what would you write about?

Come closer to me.

Press your ear against my chest, just above the whorl-lined sternum, right where the bone protrudes in an anxious knot at the center of my chest. That space is called the angle of Louis. Isn't that a lovely name? It will work best if you hold your breath while we do this. You will have to listen past the boasting of my healthy heart, past the admission of air into these working lungs, past the downbeat of my pulse. Have you arrived? Can you pick up the faint static? Yes, I agree. It does sound like a radio caught between frequencies. Like a motor on high speed. Like the echo of hope.

You found it. That's the grinding tumbler of chronic pain.

No, you can't touch it. It is not organ or nerve or blood, not bone, not entirely heart, not entirely head. Yes, it hurts. Yes, I feel it always. I know, it makes me sad, too.

I gave it a name. I created its story.

You get to tell your story, too.

How much pain can you handle? *Soon.* You found it. Cerulean. Needles in my hands, needles in my feet. Words belong. An unkindness of ravens. *Soon.* No. That's not how it happened. *I know you want answers.* Don't worry, little bird. I will touch you. How much pain can you handle? *Tuck your chin.* Split in two. Change the question. I want a word. I have proof. Yellow wax beans still firm. Incarnadine. A murmuration of starlings. I part my lips. *Soon.*

Notes

vii: *The body is not mute, but it is inarticulate.* Arthur W. Frank, *The Wounded Storyteller: Body, Illness, and Ethics* (Chicago: University of Chicago Press, 1995), 27.

2: *Use the skin swabs and antiseptic solution . . .* "Lumbar Puncture Technique," Medscape, accessed June 1, 2017, emedicine.medscape.com/article/80773-technique.

3: *He no longer instructs me to hold still, for I have become more statue than woman.* I identify as a cisgender woman. Throughout this book, I reference "woman," "women," and "female" because I am writing primarily about my own experience as a self-identified woman, but I also use these identifiers to reflect the binary lens through which medicine and history frame gender. I use this language with the full awareness that there are many who have female sex organs but do not identify as women and there are people who do not have female sex organs who identify as women. By sharing my story, I hope to expose the inequality of knowledge, care, and treatment when it comes to pain as it pertains to all people, but most especially to those whose bodies have been subjected to inadequate care.

7: *We tell ourselves stories in order to live.* Joan Didion, *The White Album* (New York: Farrar, Straus and Giroux, 1979), 11.

18: *Everyone who is born holds dual citizenship . . .* Susan Sontag, *Illness as Metaphor* (New York: Farrar, Straus and Giroux, 1977), 3.

18: *My point is that illness is* not *a metaphor . . .* Susan Sontag, *Illness as Metaphor* (New York: Farrar, Straus and Giroux, 1977), 3.

19: *the healthiest way of being ill . . .* Susan Sontag, *Illness as Metaphor* (New York: Farrar, Straus and Giroux, 1977), 3.

20: *we tell ourselves stories in order to live . . .* Joan Didion, *The White Album* (New York: Farrar, Straus and Giroux, 1979), 11.

20: *Nothing was left of Echo but her voice . . .* Ingri and Edgar Parin D'Aulaires, *Book of Greek Myths* (New York: Dell Publishing, 1962), 92.

20: *The moment she opened the lid . . .* Ingri and Edgar Parin D'Aulaires, *Book of Greek Myths* (New York: Dell Publishing, 1962), 74.

20: *At night his immortal liver grew anew* . . . Ingri and Edgar Parin D'Aulaires, *Book of Greek Myths* (New York: Dell Publishing, 1962), 72.

26: *Our show today in three acts* . . . Ira Glass, *This American Life*, Episode 325, "Houses of Ill Repute," February 2, 2007.

27: Vocabulary Lessons: Paradox. *Oxford English Dictionary*. 3rd ed. (Oxford: Oxford University Press, 2005), s.v. "Paradox."

35: *It is impossible to speak of being* . . . Paul Tillich, *Systematic Theology* (Chicago: University of Chicago Press, 1951), 181.

35: *What does experience by participation reveal* . . . Paul Tillich, *Systematic Theology* (Chicago: University of Chicago Press, 1951), 45.

35: *For that which concerns us ultimately* . . . Paul Tillich, *Systematic Theology* (Chicago: University of Chicago Press, 1951), 21.

35: *Our ultimate concern is that which determines* . . . Paul Tillich, *Systematic Theology* (Chicago: University of Chicago Press, 1951), 14.

35: *Every part is dependent on every other part* . . . Paul Tillich, *Systematic Theology* (Chicago: University of Chicago Press, 1951), 11.

36: *Nothing can be of ultimate concern* . . . Paul Tillich, *Systematic Theology* (Chicago: University of Chicago Press, 1951), 14.

36: *Providence is a paradoxical concept.* Paul Tillich, *Systematic Theology* (Chicago: University of Chicago Press, 1951), 264.

37: Vocabulary Lessons: Providence. *Oxford English Dictionary*. 3rd ed. (Oxford: Oxford University Press, 2007), s.v. "Providence."

44: *Providence is a paradoxical concept.* Paul Tillich, *Systematic Theology* (Chicago: University of Chicago Press, 1951), 264.

51: *If you wish to make an apple pie from scratch* . . . Carl Sagan, *Cosmos* (New York: Random House, 1980), 242.

53: *To have pain is to have certainty* . . . Elaine Scarry, *The Body in Pain: The Making and Unmaking of the World* (New York: Oxford University Press, 1985), 58.

55: *Arrange the pieces that come your way* . . . Anne Olivier Bell, ed., *The Diary of Virginia Woolf: Volume Three 1925–1930* (New York: Harcourt Brace Jovanovich, 1980), 39.

65: *Pain is an unpleasant sensory and emotional experience* . . . "Terminology: Pain," International Association for the Study of Pain, accessed May 23, 2023, https://www.iasp-pain.org/resources/terminology/.

67: *striking and evocative names for new concepts* ... Loren Graham and Jean-
Michel Kantor, *Naming Infinity: A True Story of Religious Mysticism and
Mathematical Creativity* (Cambridge, MA: Harvard University Press, 2009),
100.

69: *Words belong to each other.* "Words Fail Me," Virginia Woolf, first broadcast
by the BBC on April 29, 1937, as part of a series called *Words Fail Me.*
https://www.bbc.com/culture/article/20160324-the-only-surviving
-recording-of-virginia-woolf.

73: *Illness is an enemy attacker* ... Diane Nicholls, "What We Talk About When
We Talk About Illness." *MED Magazine,* Issue 15, January 2004, http://
macmillandictionaries.com/MED-Magazine/January2004/15-metaphor
-illness-print.htm. The italicized words in this passage are direct quotations
from "What We Talk About When We Talk About Illness." However, the
metaphors discussed are common.

78: Vocabulary Lessons: Patient. *Oxford English Dictionary.* 3rd ed. (Oxford:
Oxford University Press, 2005), s.v. "Patient."

81: Vocabulary Lessons: Hysteria. *Oxford English Dictionary.* 3rd ed. (Oxford:
Oxford University Press, 2020), s.v. "Hysteria."

82: *freed the emerging science from the chains of superstition* ... Helen King,
Hysteria Beyond Freud (Berkeley: University of California Press, 1993), 3.

82: *the womb is the origin of all diseases* ... Andrew Scull, *Hysteria: The Disturbing
History* (Oxford: Oxford University Press, 2009), 12.

83: *an animal within the animal* ... Helen King, *Hysteria Beyond Freud* (Berkeley:
University of California Press, 1993), 118.

84: *disease of civilization* ... Gabrielle Jackson, *Pain and Prejudice: How the
Medical System Ignores Women—and What We Can Do About It* (Vancouver,
Canada: Greystone Books, 2021), 90.

84: the *ill-defined conditions such as the vapors* ... Gabrielle Jackson, *Pain and
Prejudice: How the Medical System Ignores Women—and What We Can Do
About It* (Vancouver, Canada: Greystone Books, 2021), 92.

85: *in no small part because of their claims to own the treatment* ... Gabrielle
Jackson, *Pain and Prejudice: How the Medical System Ignores Women—and
What We Can Do About It* (Vancouver, Canada: Greystone Books, 2021), 95.

85: *while madness or lunacy wasn't yet gendered as a diagnosis* ... Gabrielle
Jackson, *Pain and Prejudice: How the Medical System Ignores Women—and
What We Can Do About It* (Vancouver, Canada: Greystone Books, 2021), 95.

85: *sexually diseased and morally debauched female imagination* . . . Helen King, *Hysteria Beyond Freud* (Berkeley: University of California Press, 1993), 185.

91: *Male-unless-otherwise* . . . Caroline Criado Perez, *Invisible Women: Data Bias in a World Designed for Men* (New York: Abrams Press, 2019), 3.

91: *turned outside in* . . . Caroline Criado Perez, *Invisible Women: Data Bias in a World Designed for Men* (New York: Abrams Press, 2019), 196.

91: *vital heat* . . . Caroline Criado Perez, *Invisible Women: Data Bias in a World Designed for Men* (New York: Abrams Press, 2019), 197.

91: *a mutilated male* . . . Caroline Criado Perez, *Invisible Women: Data Bias in a World Designed for Men* (New York: Abrams Press, 2019), 196.

91: *the prevalence, course and severity of the majority of common human diseases* . . . Caroline Criado Perez, *Invisible Women: Data Bias in a World Designed for Men* (New York: Abrams Press, 2019), 198.

92: *fluctuating, "atypical" hormones* . . . Caroline Criado Perez, *Invisible Women: Data Bias in a World Designed for Men* (New York: Abrams Press, 2019), 202.

97: Data Collection: Beck Depression Inventory. "Beck Depression Inventory," https://www.ohsu.edu/sites/default/files/2019-06/Beck%20 Depression%20Inventory.pdf.

114: *The law is on the side of the normal.* Virginia Woolf, *On Being Ill* (Ashfield, MA: Paris Press; Reprint edition, 2012), 23.

123: *just as faithful, just as obtrusive and shameless, just as entertaining, just as clever* . . . Friedrich Nietzsche, *The Gay Science.* 1st ed. (1882), trans. Walter Kaufmann (New York: Vintage Press, 1974), 249–50.

131: *Anger is the single, most salient emotional contributor to pain.* Soraya Chemaly, *Rage Becomes Her: The Power of Women's Anger* (New York: Atria Books, 2018), 51.

131: *Scientists have found that the stronger the curse words* . . . Soraya Chemaly, *Rage Becomes Her: The Power of Women's Anger* (New York: Atria Books, 2018), 52.

131: *Cursing numbs pain* . . . Soraya Chemaly, *Rage Becomes Her: The Power of Women's Anger* (New York: Atria Books, 2018), 52.

132: *Women in pain are often women enraged* . . . Soraya Chemaly, *Rage Becomes Her: The Power of Women's Anger* (New York: Atria Books, 2018), 52.

135: *the poverty of the language* . . . Virginia Woolf, *On Being Ill* (Ashfield, MA: Paris Press; Reprint edition, 2012), 6.

136: *I want to write rage but all that comes is sadness.* Audre Lorde, *The Cancer Journals* (New York: Penguin Books, 1980), 5.

137: The McGill Pain Questionnaire. Ronald Melzack and Warren S. Torgerson, "On the Language of Pain," *Anesthesiology* 34 (January 1971): 50–59.

139: *not only a new language that we need* ... Virginia Woolf, *On Being Ill* (Ashfield, MA: Paris Press; Reprint edition, 2012), 7.

140: *Words belong to each other.* "Words Fail Me," Virginia Woolf, first broadcast by the BBC on April 29, 1937, as part of a series called *Words Fail Me.* https://www.bbc.com/culture/article/20160324-the-only-surviving -recording-of-virginia-woolf.

147: *There is a childish outspokenness in illness* ... Virginia Woolf, *On Being Ill* (Ashfield, MA: Paris Press; Reprint edition, 2012), 11.

147: *Illness is the great confessional.* Virginia Woolf, *On Being Ill* (Ashfield, MA: Paris Press; Reprint edition, 2012), 11.

147: *All day, all night the body intervenes.* Virginia Woolf, *On Being Ill* (Ashfield, MA: Paris Press; Reprint edition, 2012), 4.

147: *The body smashes itself to smithereens* ... Virginia Woolf, *On Being Ill* (Ashfield, MA: Paris Press; Reprint edition, 2012), 5.

148: *To look these things squarely in the face would need the courage of a lion tamer.* Virginia Woolf, *On Being Ill* (Ashfield, MA: Paris Press; Reprint edition, 2012), 5.

148: *A reason rooted in the bowels of the earth.* Virginia Woolf, *On Being Ill* (Ashfield, MA: Paris Press; Reprint edition, 2012), 5.

155: *A wound marks the threshold between interior and exterior.* Leslie Jamison, *The Empathy Exams* (Minneapolis: Graywolf Press, 2014), 194.

159: *mere transaction of the nervous system.* David Norris, *The Culture of Pain* (Berkeley: University of California Press, 1991), 20.

188: *sick and yet happy, in peril and yet happy* ... Bertrand Russell, *A History of Western Philosophy* (New York: Taylor and Francis, 2004), 251.

206: *man writ large.* Fergus Kerr, "Cartesianism According to Karl Barth," *New Blackfriars* 77, no. 906 (August 1996): 358–68.

216: *Pain comes from the darkness* ... Randall Jarrell, "90 North," *The Complete Poems* (New York: Farrar, Straus and Giroux, 1969), 114.

228: The Visual Analogue Scale. M. H. Hayes. "Experimental Development of the Graphic Rating Method." *Psychological Bulletin* 18 (1921): 98–99.

230: *The pain scale measures only the intensity of pain, not the duration.* Eula Biss, "The Pain Scale." *Harper's Magazine*, June 2005.

230: *A measure of pain, I believe, requires at least two dimensions* . . . Eula Biss, "The Pain Scale." *Harper's Magazine,* June 2005.

232: *dol* . . . *perceptible steps in discrimination of stimulus intensity* . . . C. Ball and R. N. Westhorpe, "The History of Pain Measurement," *Anaesthesia and Intensive Care* 39, no. 4 (July 2011): 529.

232: *the dolorimeter may have application* . . . C. Ball and R. N. Westhorpe, "The History of Pain Measurement," *Anaesthesia and Intensive Care* 39, no. 4 (July 2011): 529.

233: *account all the subjective, emotional overlays* . . . C. Ball and R. N. Westhorpe, "The History of Pain Measurement," *Anaesthesia and Intensive Care* 39, no. 4 (July 2011): 529.

234: *The pain experience has three components.* Fernando Cervero, *Understanding Pain: Exploring the Perception of Pain* (Cambridge, MA: MIT Press, 2012), 88.

236: Notions of "monster" and "miracle" are taken from Virginia Woolf, *On Being Ill* (Paris Press; Reprint edition, 2012), 6.

239: *The pain experience has three components.* Fernando Cervero, *Understanding Pain: Exploring the Perception of Pain* (Cambridge, MA: MIT Press, 2012), 88.

240: *the brotherhood of those who bear the mark of pain.* Albert Schweitzer, *Out of My Life and Thought: An Autobiography.* Trans. Antje Bultmann Lemke (1993, New York: Henry Holt, 1990), 195.

242: *The body is not mute, but it is inarticulate.* Arthur W. Frank, *The Wounded Storyteller: Body, Illness, and Ethics* (Chicago: University of Chicago Press, 1995), 27.

251: *New daily persistent headaches come on suddenly* . . . "Chronic Daily Headaches," Mayo Clinic, accessed June 22, 2018. mayoclinic.org/diseases-conditions/chronic-daily-headaches/symptoms-causes/syc-20370891.

252: *Providence is a paradoxical concept.* Paul Tillich, *Systematic Theology* (Chicago: University of Chicago Press, 1951), 264.

255: *I had never wanted to be right, only to be well.* From *Ask Me About My Uterus* by Abby Norman, copyright © 2018. Reprinted by permission of Bold Type Books, an imprint of Hachette Book Group, Inc.

271: *Did you know the Spanish word for waiting and hoping is the same* . . . Rabih Alameddine, *The Angel of History* (New York: Atlantic Monthly Press, 2016).

282: *Providence is a paradoxical concept.* Paul Tillich, *Systematic Theology* (Chicago: University of Chicago Press, 1951), 264.

296: *Whatever pain achieves, it achieves in part through its unsharability* ... Elaine Scarry, *The Body in Pain: The Making and Unmaking of the World* (New York: Oxford University Press, 1985), 4.

Acknowledgments

ENTERTAINING PAIN as a subject is one thing. Exposing personal pain is quite another. It requires a peculiar mix of empathy and persistence to continually support those who live with irreconcilable, unpredictable pain. Because of this, I am humbled by those who have earned the right to stand next to my most vulnerable self and those who have stepped in to support my creative efforts.

With gratitude, I would like to thank the exceptionally talented crew at the University of Iowa Press, including Susan Hill Newton, Meredith Stabel, Allison Means, and James McCoy. To Nicole Wayland. To Kathleen Lynch. To Jordan Kisner and Abby Norman, who put their shoulders behind this unconventional book.

Perhaps more than anyone else, Rachel Yoder, Alisha Jeddeloh, and Jennifer Colville coaxed this book into being. With compassion and curiosity, they encouraged this story to take up more space. What a privilege to write in such splendid company.

I am grateful for the bevy of friends, family, colleagues, and fellow artists whose lives and creative work have been present fixtures throughout this project. Thank you for asking the exact right questions. Thank you for listening to my answers. Thank you to my co-editors at *Brink* who understand that broken bodies tell broken stories.

I want to acknowledge the many doctors, nurses, clinicians, and therapists who have offered tremendously skilled guidance, gentle care, and steady direction throughout this tangled experience. To those who live in the land of in-between: I see you and I'm so sorry we're here. Let's harness our power to instigate change.

To my parents, Dave Lohman and Sherry Lohman, who nurture with unparalleled capacity and generosity. Thank you for providing support without question or condition. To my sisters, Beth and Michelle, and their families, Jon, Jeremiah, Sierra, Jay, Lohman, Avery, Jameson, and Finley: my wolfpack and source of adventure, food, and laughter. What luck to spend this life with you. To my co-parent, Joe Cilek, who witnessed the dismantling and has participated in the rebuilding of this crooked life.

And lastly, thank you to my children, Adel and Ezra, whose lives, by extension and exposure, are shaped by the presence of pain. I am astounded by your adaptability. Your grace and humor and tenderness are the stuff of dreams. I love you.